Tomita
— method —
JAPANESE OSTEOPATHY

EFFICIENT MYOFASCIA RELEASE
PROFESSIONAL COURSE MANUAL

BY NORIO TOMITA

EFFICIENT MYOFASCIA RELEASE
PROFESSIONAL COURSE MANUAL

Atelier Tomita
October 2017

Conceived by Norio Tomita, CEO, Atelier Tomita
Designed and Edited by Christine Lavoie-Gagnon
Published by CLAGA
ISBN: 978-1-989021-00-2

DISCLAIMER

www.ateliertomita.com

PURPOSE OF THIS COURSE

1. To understand the inter-connection of myofascial tension around the body

2. To master 2 types of hand techniques for releasing body tension

3. To learn the points to treat in order to release the tension

4. To master self-maintenance techniques

CONTENTS

BODY ORIENTATION

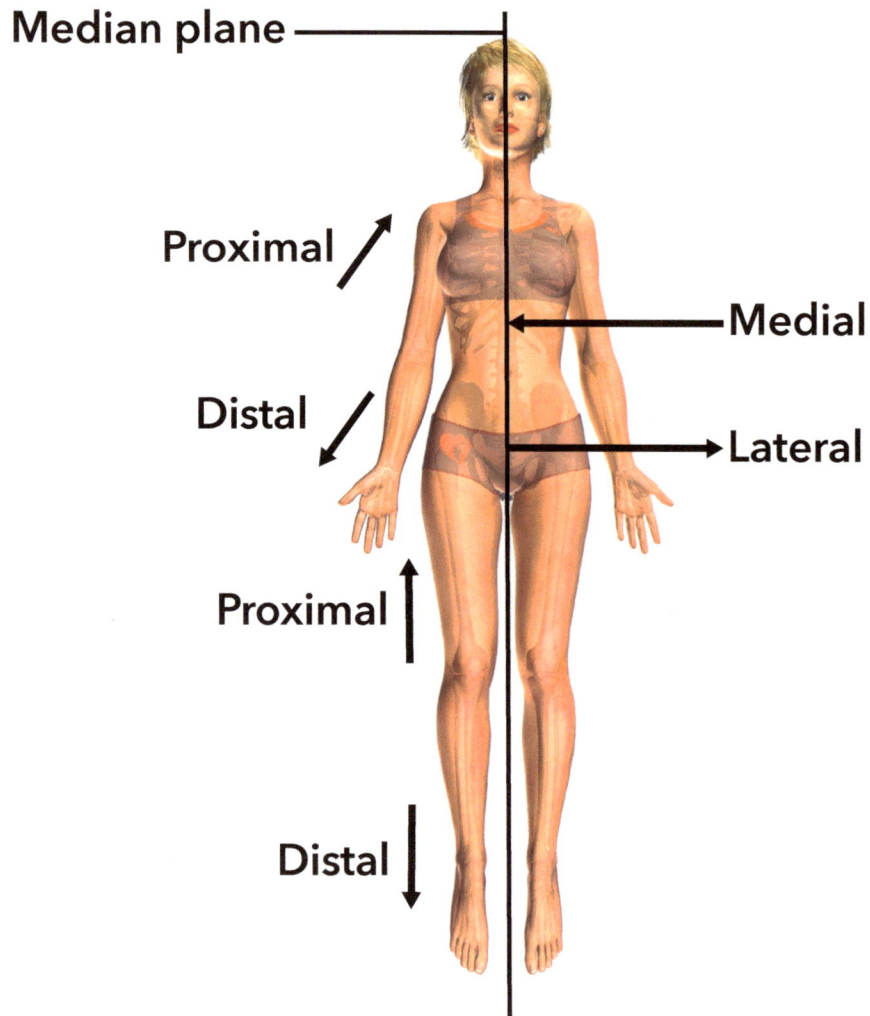

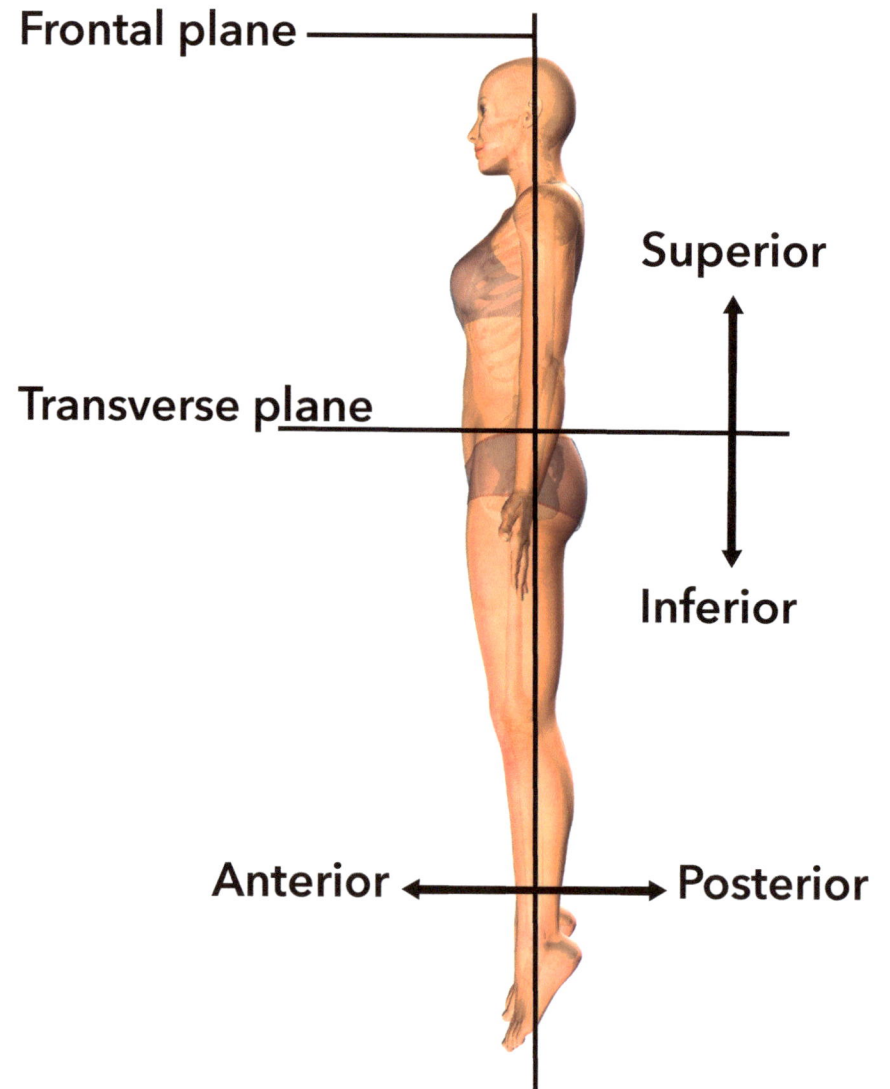

Median plane

Proximal

Distal

Medial

Lateral

Proximal

Distal

Frontal plane

Transverse plane

Superior

Inferior

Anterior

Posterior

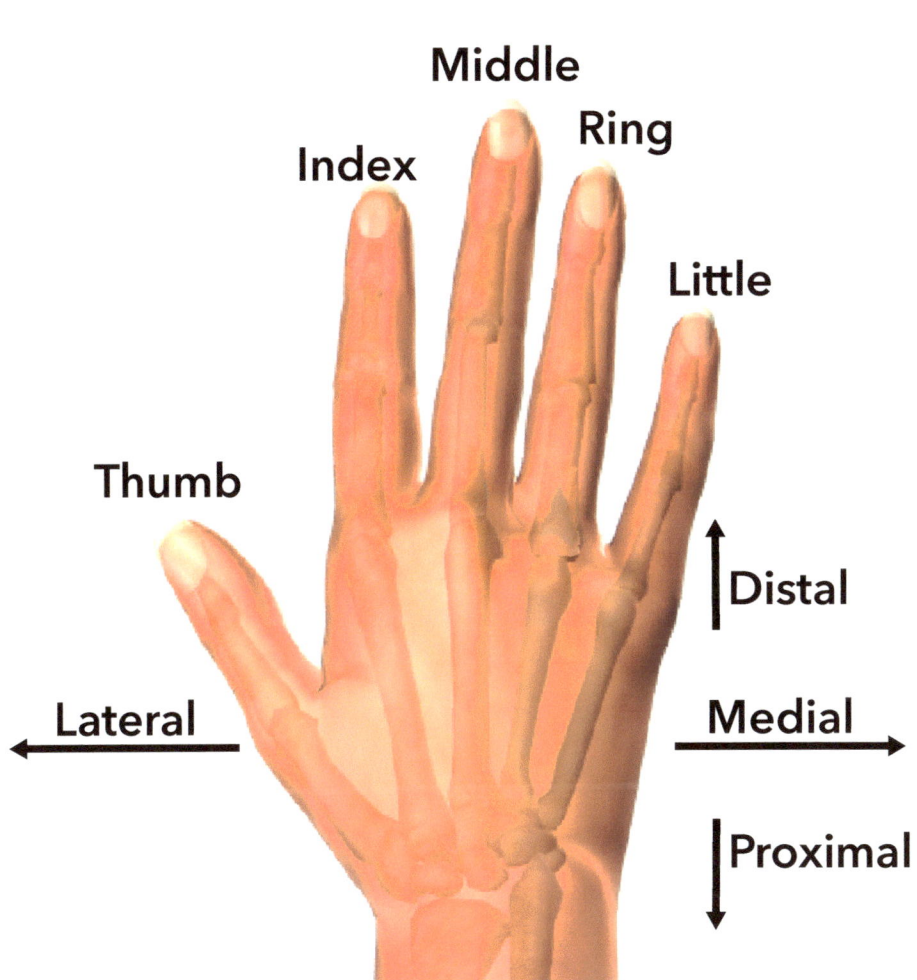

Middle

Index

Ring

Thumb

Little

Distal

Lateral

Medial

Proximal

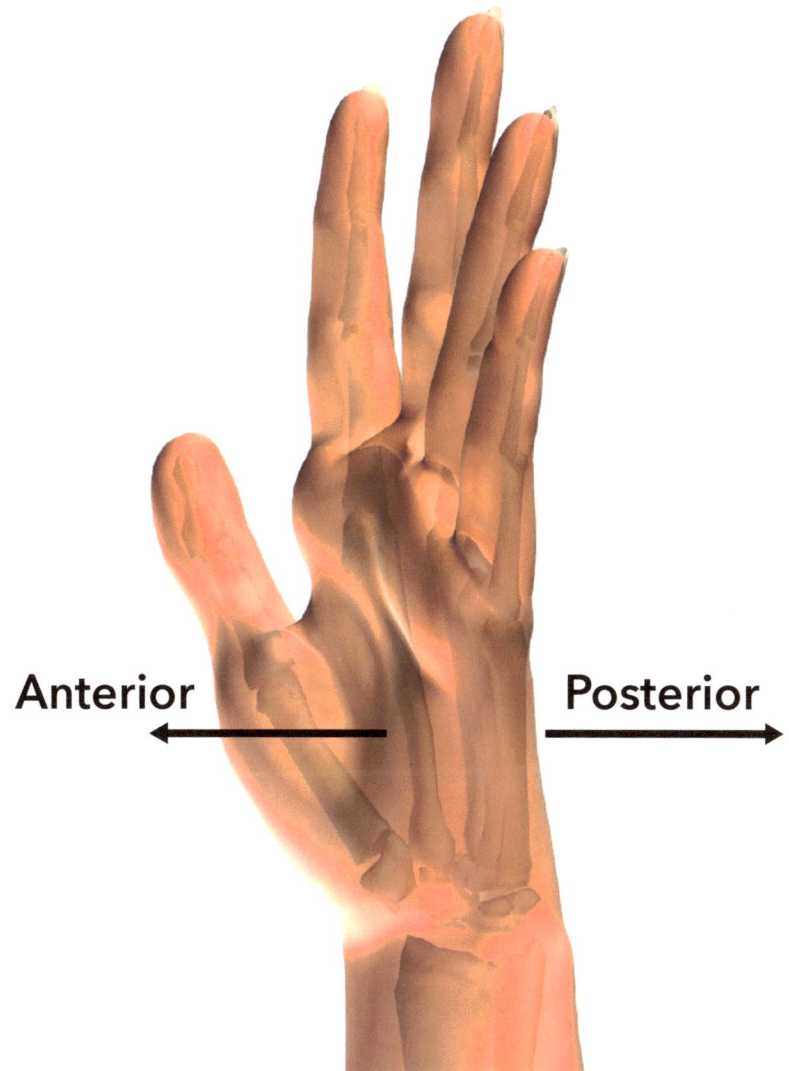

Anterior

Posterior

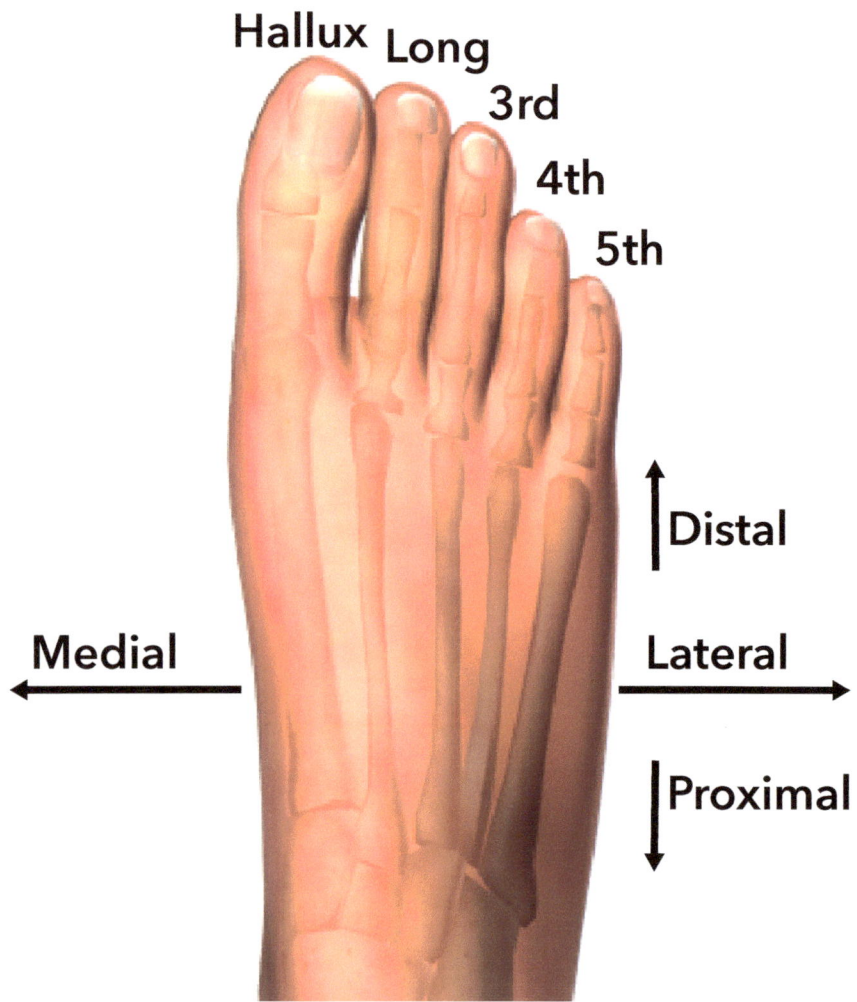

Hallux Long
3rd
4th
5th

↑ Distal

Medial ← → Lateral

↓ Proximal

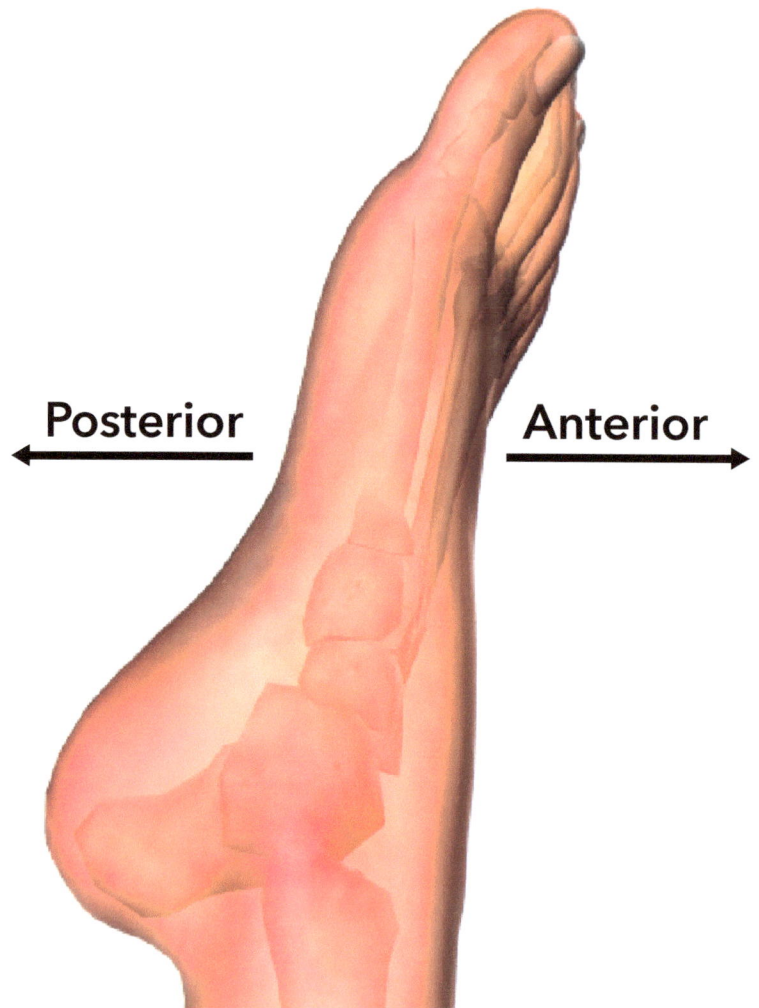

Posterior ← → Anterior

SELF MAINTENANCE TECHNIQUE

Before any session, prepare:

1. Release your diaphragm:

   - Sit on your hip bones
   - Exhale as much as you can, while leaning forward

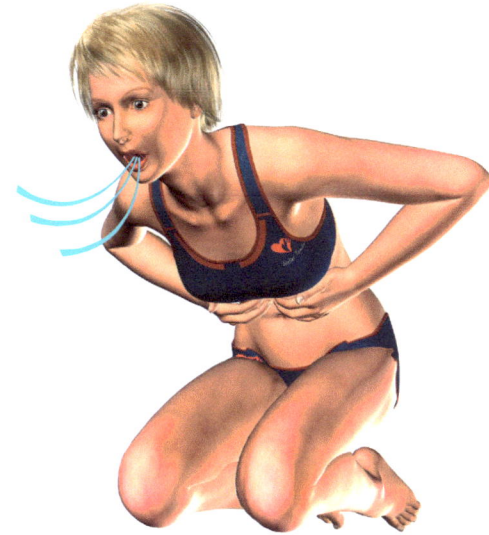

2. Light exercise to release your own body tension:

   - Spread your legs to the width of your shoulders
   - Bend your knees slightly
   - Spread your weight through the entire soles of your feet
   - Shake down your hands and follow the vibrations with your entire body
   - Never jump up
   - Never shake your hands forward

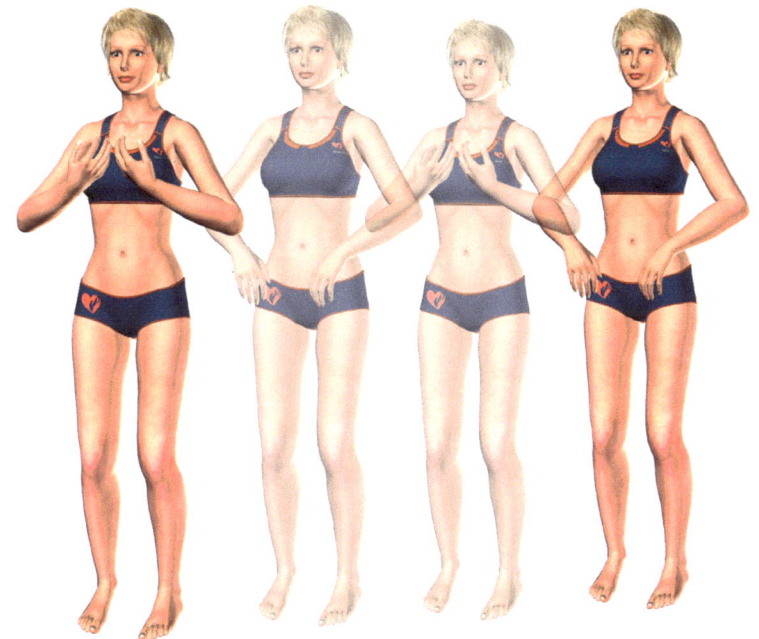

DIAGNOSIS AND HAND TECHNIQUES

OUTLINE

1. Understand the cause of Pain or Symptom
2. Two major treatment approaches based on natural body reaction:
   - Releasing skin tension
   - Soft stimulation of myofascia
3. Diagnose dominant body tension
4. Sensing myofascial tension

UNDERSTAND THE CAUSE OF PAIN OR SYMPTOM

1. In this course, we will focus on the role of myofascia in the cause of pain and body tensions. Science doesn't universally agree on the exact difference in definition between FASCIA and MYO-FASCIA. For the purpose of clarity, this book makes no distinction between the two and will only use the word MYOFASCIA.

2. Myofascia is the thin white tissue extending from the tendon, that encapsulates all muscles and internal organs. It contains tiny sensory nerves that communicate to the brain. You can think of it as a protective net that holds everything together in the body.

3. Muscle tension of a certain body part is connected to the entire body. Our bodies are made to distribute and mitigate tension. This means if you hurt one foot, your whole body provides support to compensate a weakened area, so you keep balance while giving some rest for the time that the hurting heals.

4. If you feel pain not related to a specific injury — tension in your lower-back for example — that pain could be the symptom of compensation for another problem located at another part of your body. It is thus important to understand the connectivities of the myofascia throughout the body in order to find the origin of the problem.

1. It is thus important not to treat only the painful area, as there might be many other compensating areas with less sensory nerves or in parts of the body that we don't usually move — along the rib cage for example.

2. When a muscle gets stiff, the myofascia and tendon stick to the bone (or the myofascia between

muscles stick together) and restrain the muscle movements, which can lead to tension, pain or inflammation. Releasing this myofascia from the bone helps to recover the flexibility of the muscle.

3. The hand technique that you will learn through this course will show you how some little stimulation on the tendon or some gentle stroke on the skin can effectively and sometimes instantly release muscle tension. These methods are very different from massage.

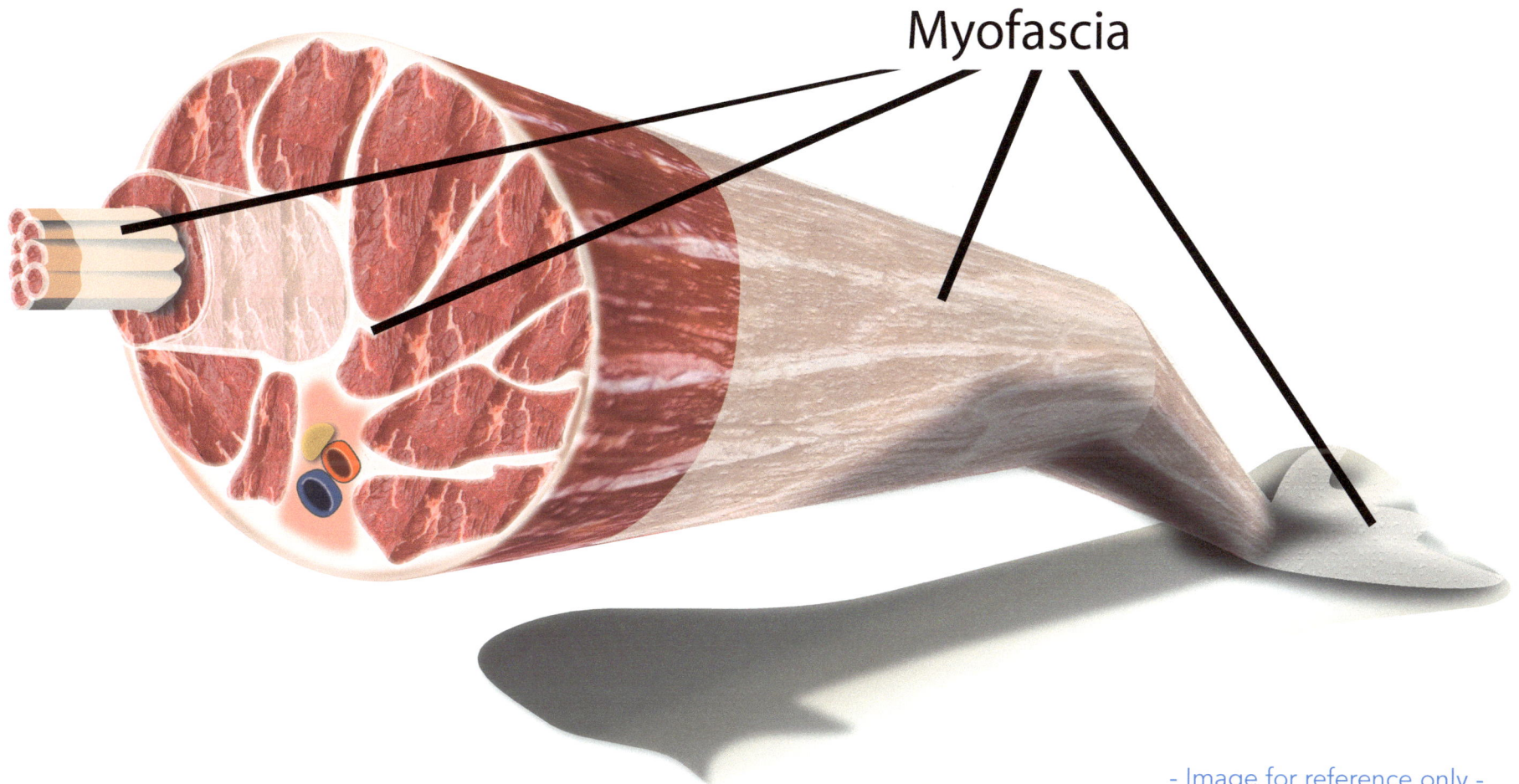

Myofascia

- Image for reference only -
See also: Anatomy Train

TWO MAJOR TREATMENT APPROACHES

1 RELEASING SKIN TENSION

Mechanism

Healthy skin moves apart from muscles and bones at surgical fascia. But around the areas where we feel pain or less joint flexibility, the skin is stiffer, and can barely be twitched.

Gentle strokes in the right direction help to recover the skin's flexibility.

Each body part has it's own skin direction for strokes, but basically, the strokes should be upward (superior direction) for anterior/medial parts of the body, and downward (inferior direction) for posterior/lateral parts of the body.

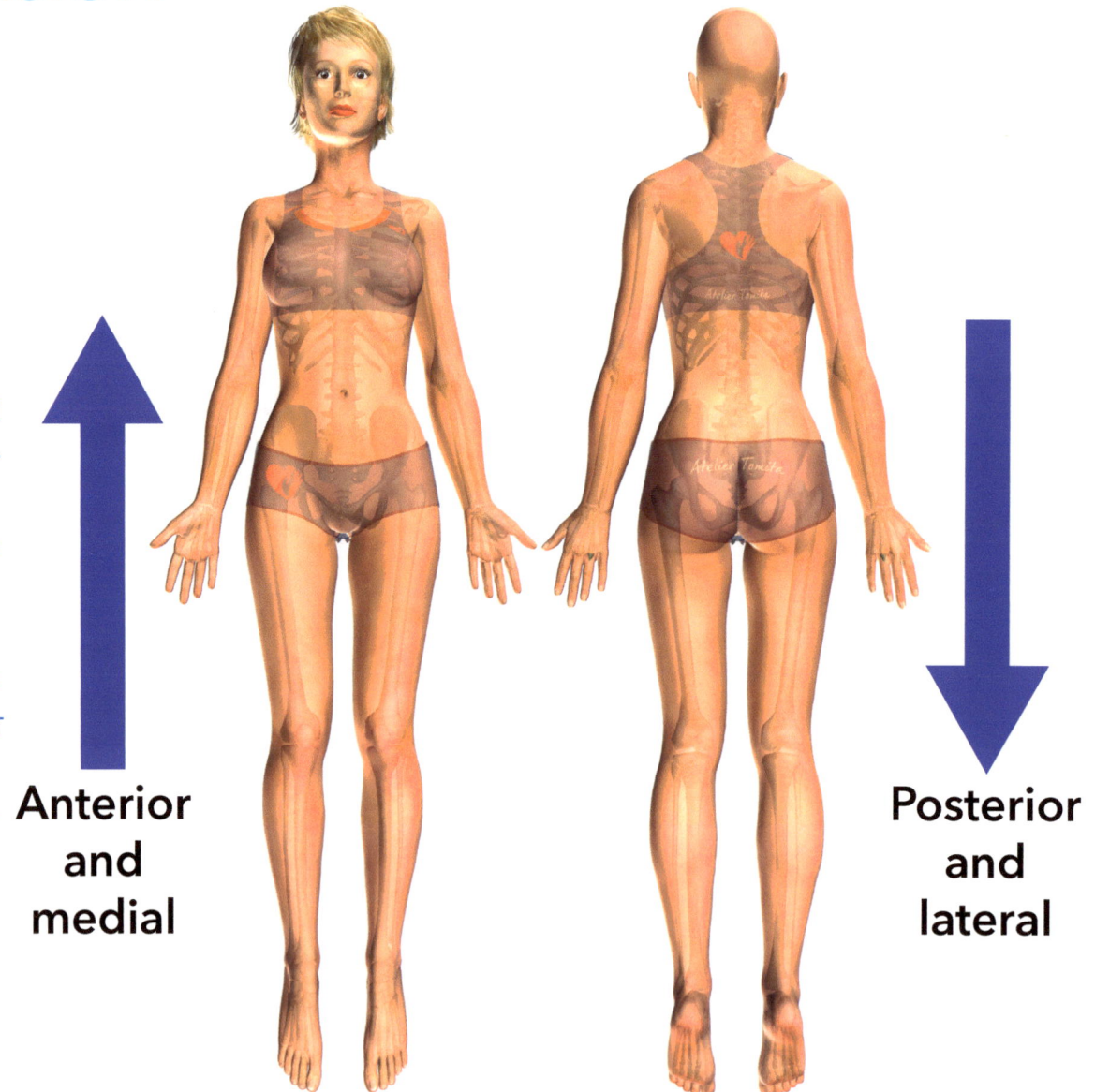

Anterior and medial

Posterior and lateral

Hand Technique: **STROKES**

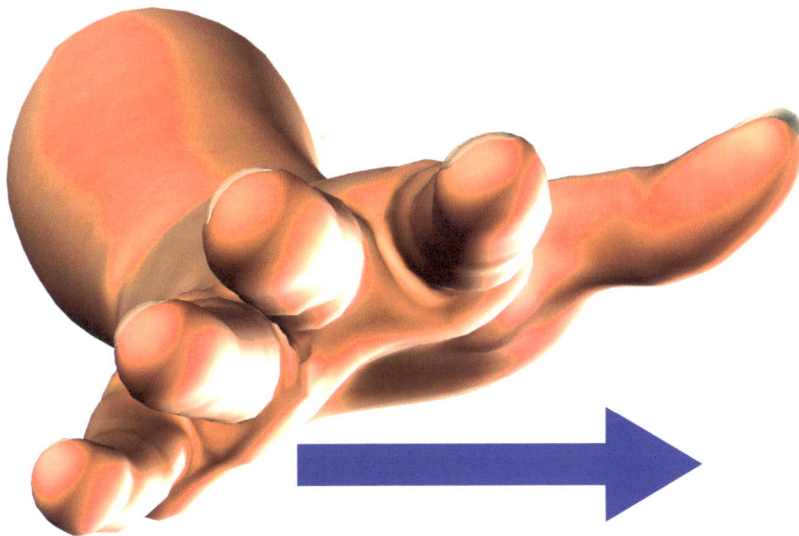

Just gently STROKE with your 4 fingers at equal strength. The ring finger is the easiest to use if you want a little more strength to the STROKE. The pressure should vary from very gentle to medium, as you would use to stroke a cat.

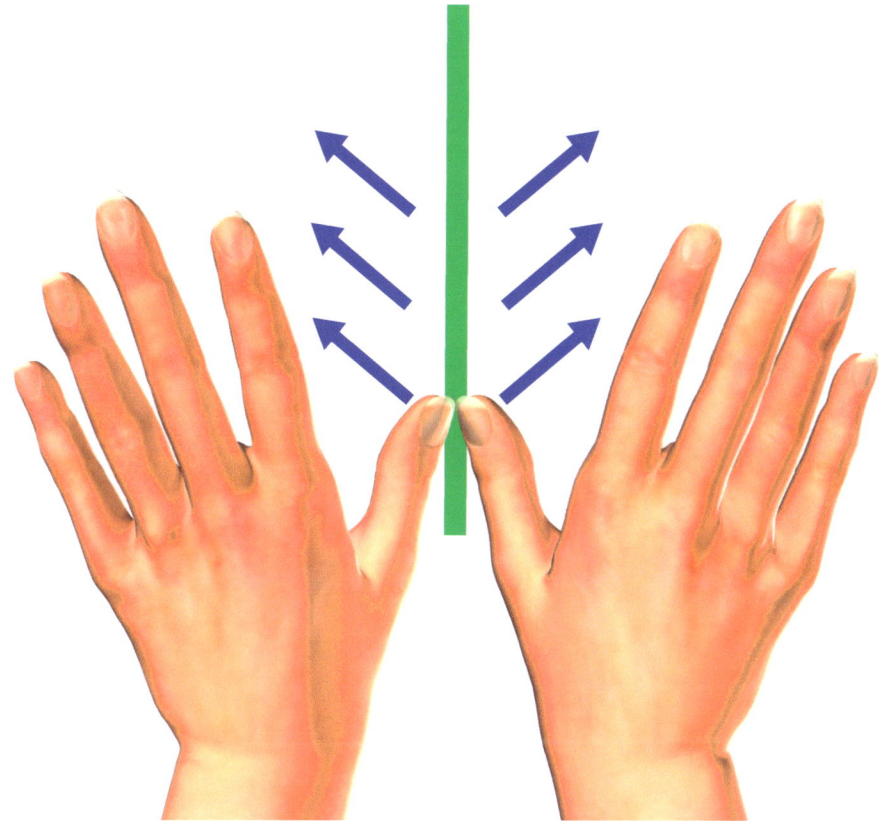

Around the convex part of a bone, thumbs are more useful to STROKE. And when releasing the skin along a tension line, STROKE as if you wanted to open the skin along the green line, as the blue arrows show.

2 SOFT STIMULATION OF MYOFASCIA

Mechanism

Myofascial connection has gained in recognition during recent years, and we are starting to understand that it is not only the muscles, but also myofascia, that contribute to the expansion of tension throughout the body, which would also explain the reason of pain.
Myofascial trigger points were found in the middle of each muscle, and the latest treatment approach is to stimulate these points to decrease the tension along myofascial connection lines.

These trigger points are the location points of felt symptom/pain, or close to them. Some Japanese techniques, however, leave the muscle untouched and the focus is set only at the edge of the underneath bone. The tension is released with gentle stimulation of these edges with the tip of the fingernail. They are located in the distal part of the body, far from the points of symptom/pain.

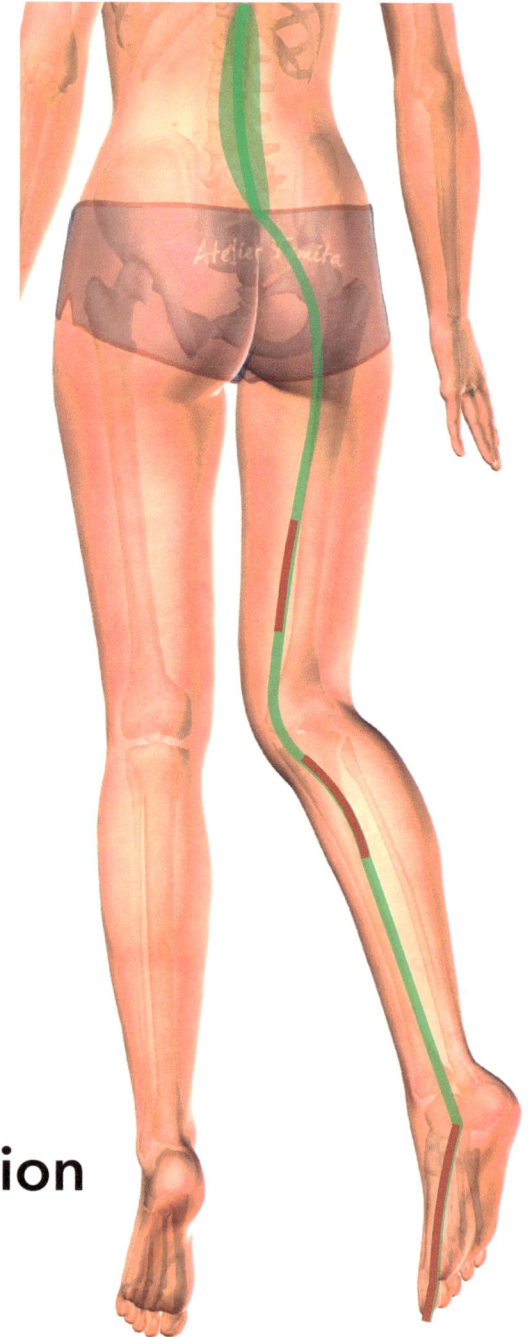

Area of pain
Myofascial connection
Point to treat

Myofascia hangs on the slope of the convex part of the bone, in a similar way we hang on wall-climbing grips. When pulled from proximal across a joint (as shown with the green line on the left picture), myofascia hangs on the bone at 3 points:

1. proximal slope of distal convex of proximal bone.
2. proximal slope of proximal slope of distal bone.
3. distal slope of proximal convex of distal bone.

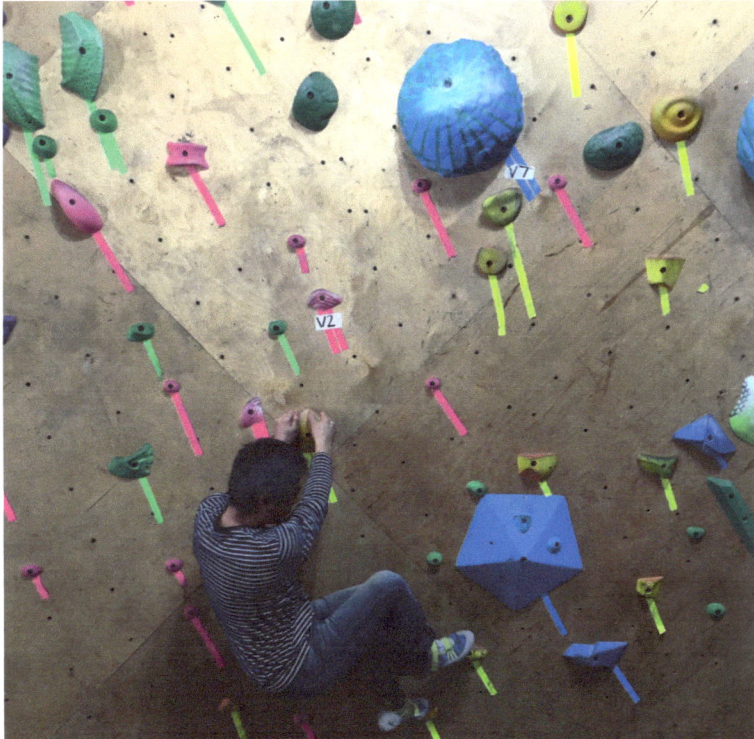

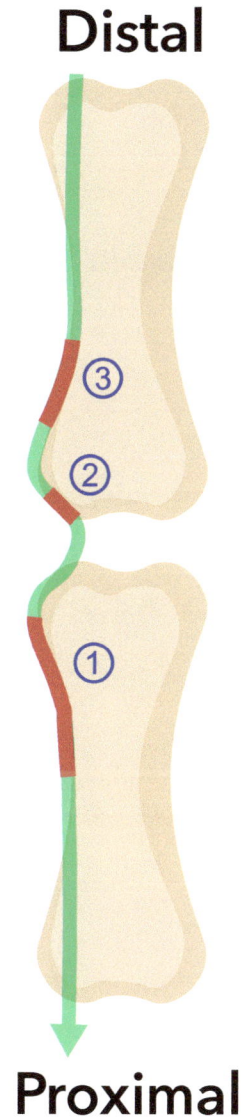

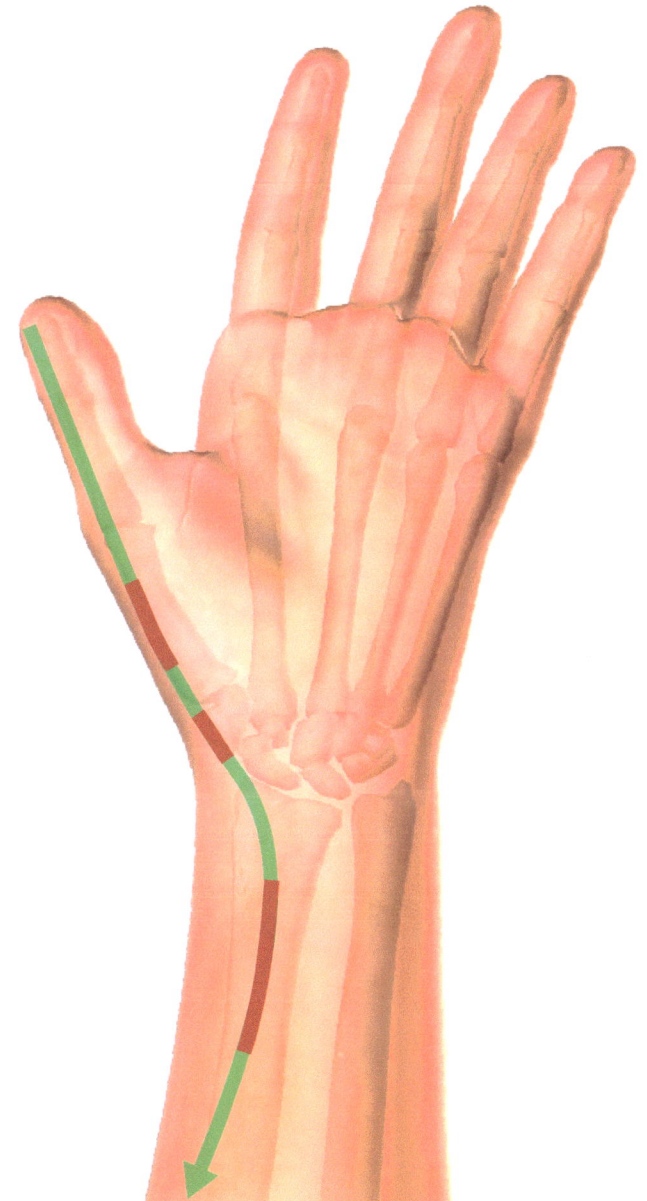

Distal

③

②

①

Proximal

Hand Technique: **SCRATCHING**

Use your nail like the edge of a knife to stimulate the bone edge. Slide swiftly but DON'T put power in your thumb. If you find the right edge of the bone, it won't be necessary to use any power. NEVER scratch the skin directly. ALWAYS do top-down movements.

File roundly after cutting your fingernails short, don't leave them jag. You can use strengthening nail polish if you have thin or weak fingernails.

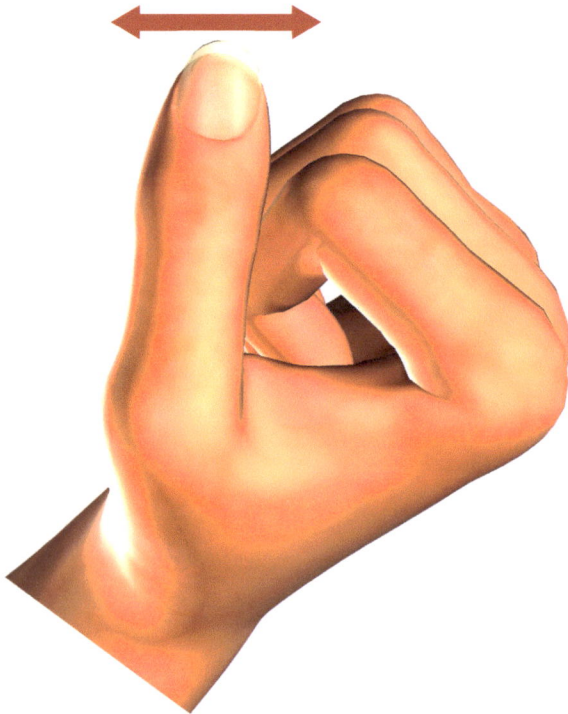

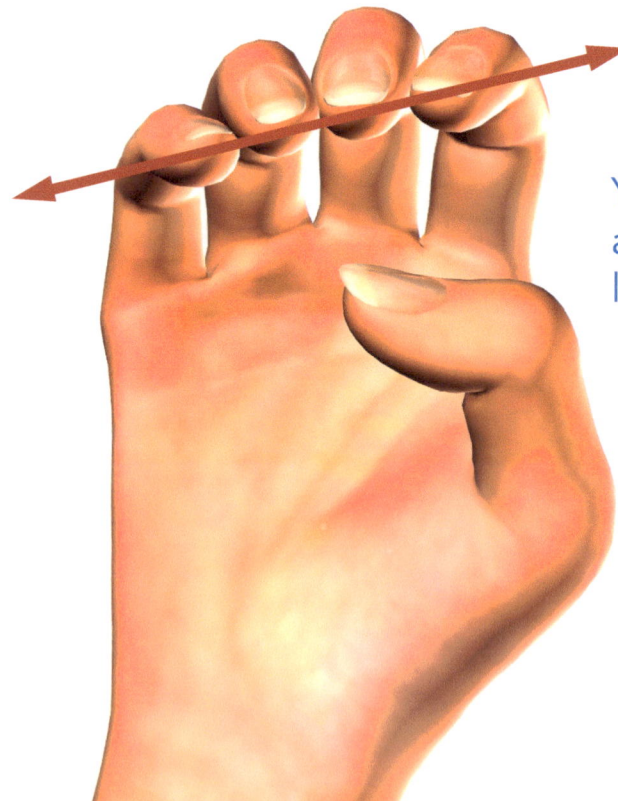

You can use 4 fingers together as one blade when you scratch longer lines.

If you have tension in your hand or if you press too hard, you might hurt your patient.

You will not be able to sense the myofascial tension either.

Hand Technique: PULLING

Sometimes you will have to pull part of the body to release myofascial stiffness. It is important to pull gently with your body weight. NEVER pull with your arm strength.

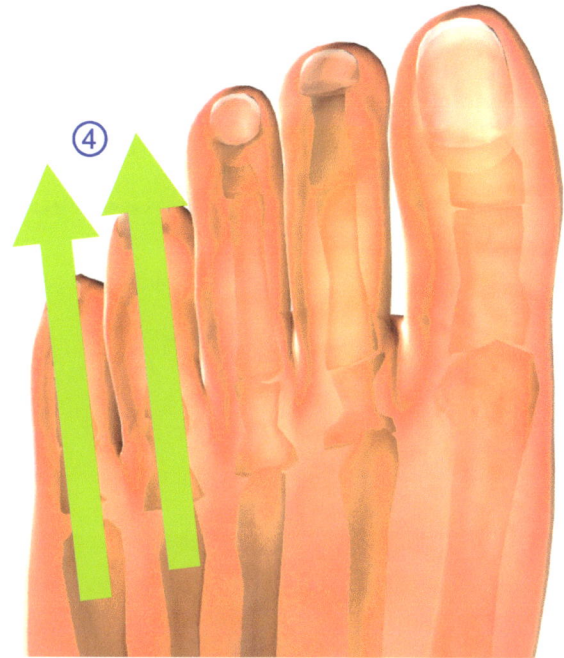

Hand Technique: SLIDING

After SCRATCHING, you will often have to SLIDE the myofascia to the side, usually perpendicular way of the bone edge. Use the palm of your hand for large areas and the tip of your fingers for smaller or thinner areas.
This also allows you to verify if your SCRATCHES were efficient or not.

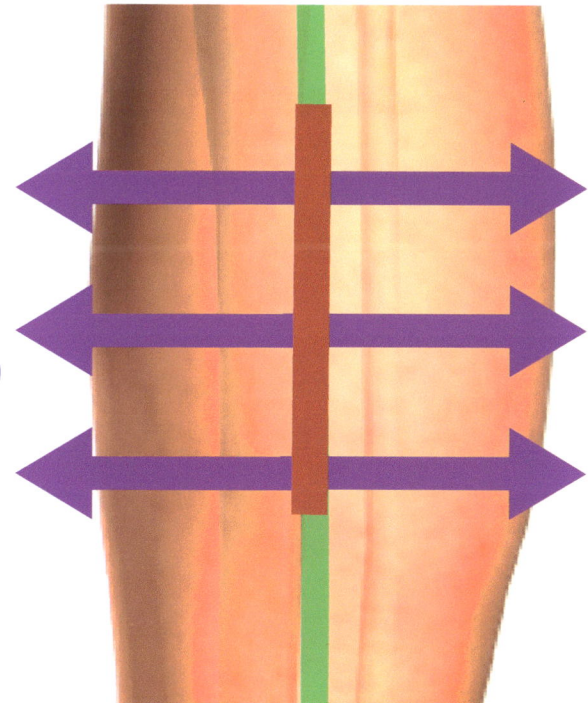

SENSING MYOFASCIAL TENSION

1. When touching your patient to verify myofascial stiffness, you must completely relax your arms, from the shoulders to the end of your finger tips.

2. Do not use pressure, but rather gentle moves with you open hands, to sense all the layers of tension inside the patient's body, from skin to muscles, to deep tissue around the bones.

3. Take your time to slowly feel which part is stiffer than others and where the myofascia seems to be tighter.

4. Start by softly moving the skin with your palm, then gradually add a little pressure to move a layer deeper.

5. When you use this hand technique properly, you will be able to feel the movement of all the layers down to the deep tissue.

If you have tension in your hand or if you press too hard, you might hurt your patient.

You will not be able to sense the myofascial tension either.

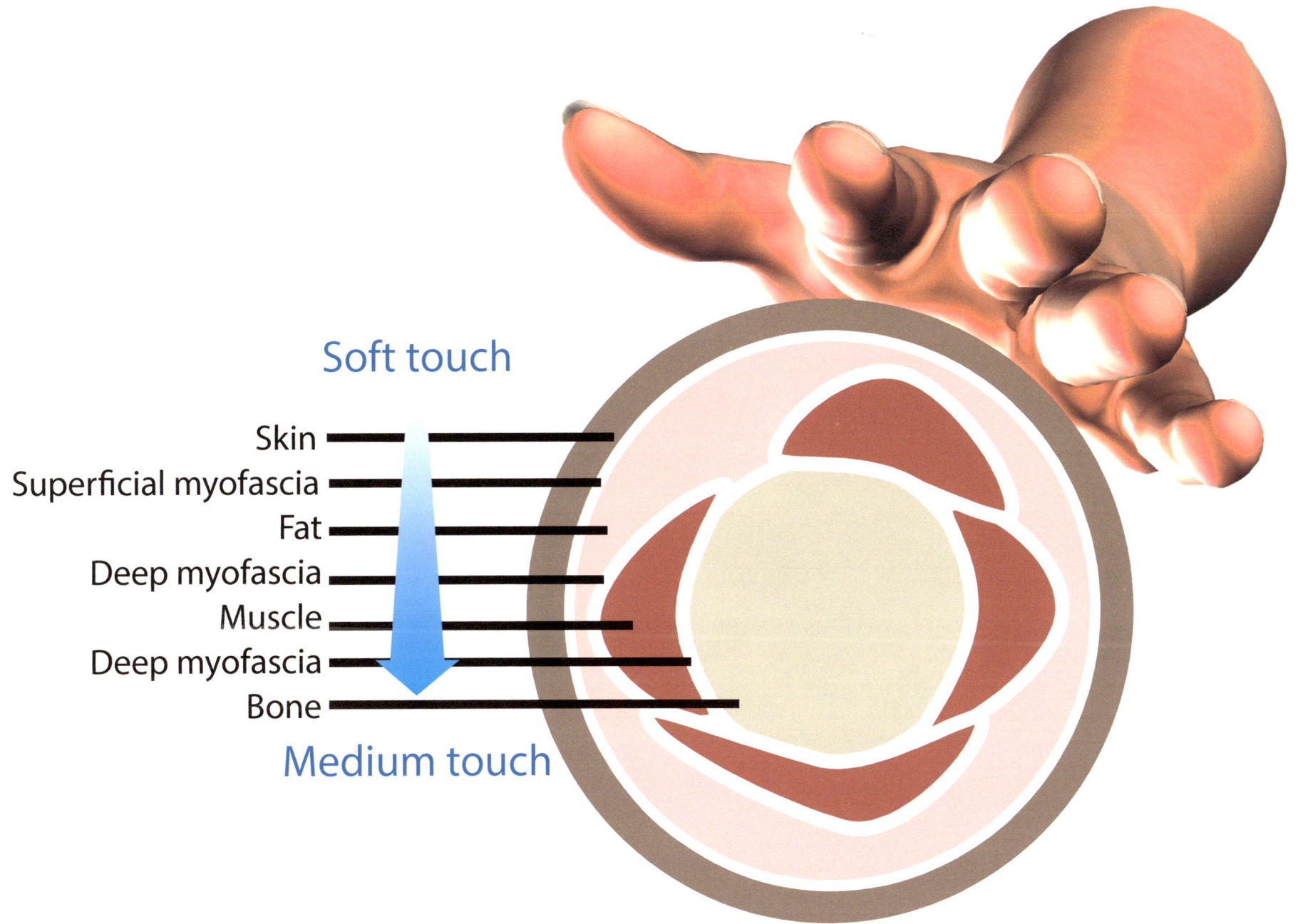

Soft touch

Skin
Superficial myofascia
Fat
Deep myofascia
Muscle
Deep myofascia
Bone

Medium touch

DIAGNOSE DOMINANT BODY TENSION

Always start a treatment session by identifying which side of the body has the dominant tension. Patients will express their pain and you can start from there to evaluate the treatment points, but you must also carefully take into account the dominant body tension.

Patients will mention the most sensitive areas of their body, but you must look for the other hidden painful points that are also affecting the chain of connective tension. Most patients will discover them as you point them out. It is very important to **release the entire body stiffness** in order to get rid of those very painful areas. Only then can the body reset to its neutral status.

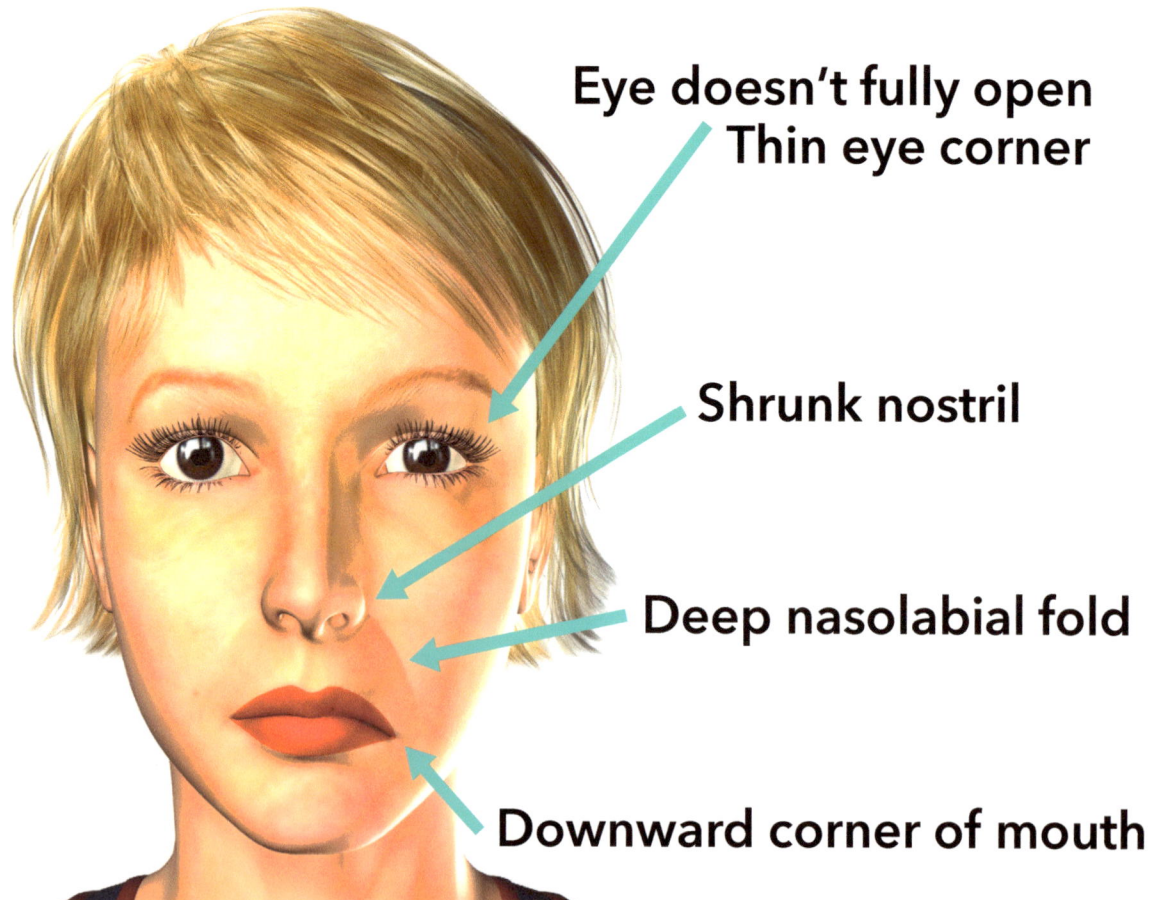

Treating only the area that the patient points out is very ineffective and can even increase inflammation of the affected tissue.

Eye doesn't fully open
Thin eye corner

Shrunk nostril

Deep nasolabial fold

Downward corner of mouth

MAJOR SIGNS INDICATING DOMINANT SIDE OF BODY TENSION

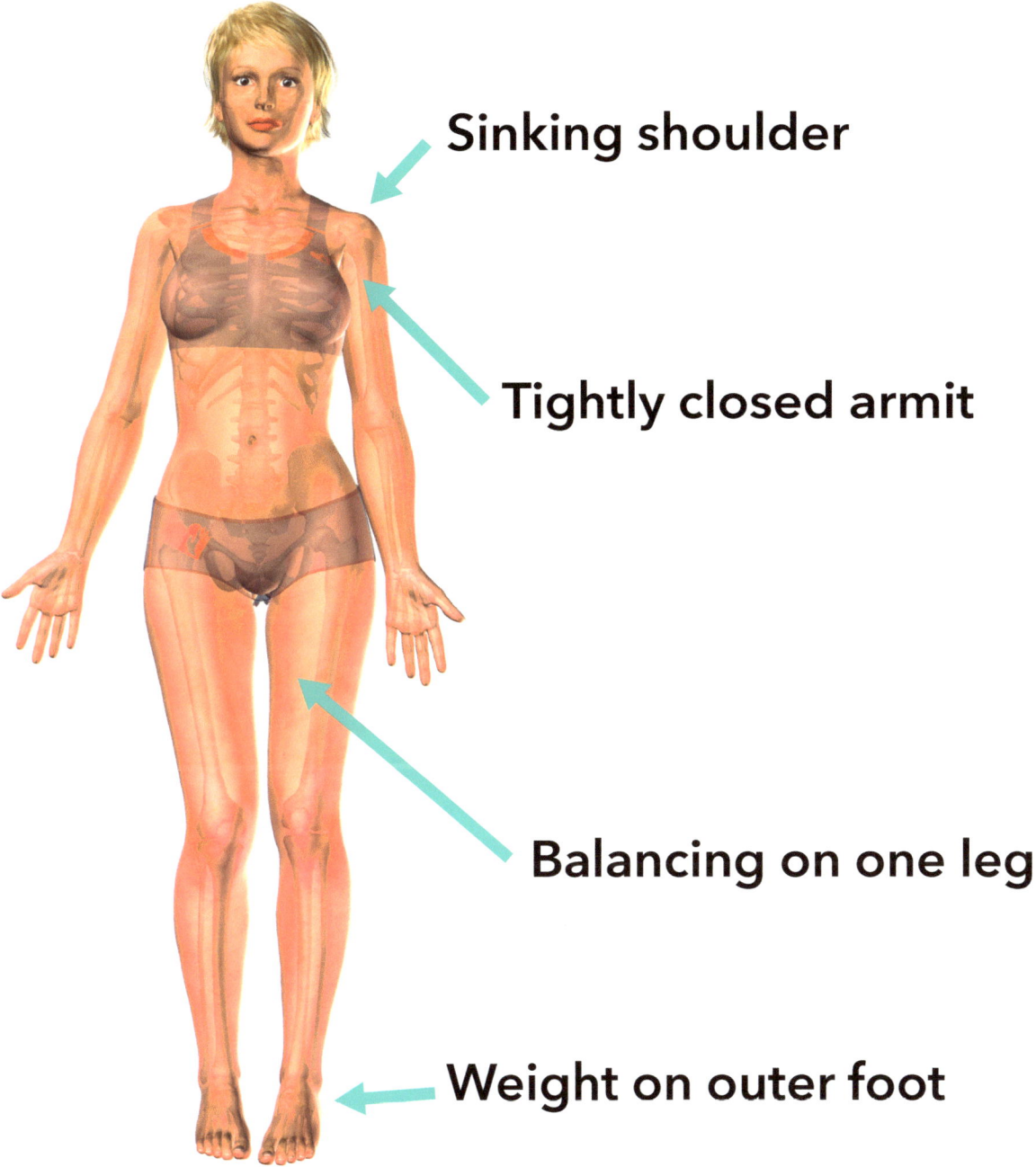

Sinking shoulder

Tightly closed armit

Balancing on one leg

Weight on outer foot

EVALUATION

1. How does myofascia work?

2. What is the difference between massage and the Tomita method?

3. What are the 2 major treatment approaches?

4. Can you perform the 2 main hand techniques?

5. Can you sense the different layers of myofascial stiffness?

6. Can you tell the dominant side of body tension ?

NOTES

RECOVERING DEEP BREATH

OUTLINE

1. Widen the nasal cavity
   - How to adjust nasal laterality and release forehead tension
2. Widen the respiratory tract
   - How to release throat tension
3. Widen the rib cage
   - How to release tension around the sternum
   - How to release tension of the diaphragm
   - How to release tension on the back of the chest
4. Self maintenance technique
   - Two ways to decrease tiredness on your own body.

WIDEN THE NASAL CAVITY

Mechanism:

A stuffy nose creates tension on the forehead, and this tension spreads along the Green Lines as seen on the picture.

⚠️ There are 2 ways of widening the nasal cavity and both can be combined. SCRATCHING is more efficient and quicker, but some patients might not like the strong feeling of it, particularly on their face. In this case, the STROKES approach should be used. It takes more time but it is very gentle.

Treatment: SCRATCHING

1. Massage the Green Point:
   Find a tiny hollow spot with your nail and massage up and down or gently pinch around it.
   (Meridian Point GV24)
2. SCRATCH down the forehead to release myo-fascia from sticking to the scalp.
3. SCRATCH right below the cheek bones

⚠️ Use a thicker cloth if you choose to SCRATCH on the face, as the skin is very delicate in this area.

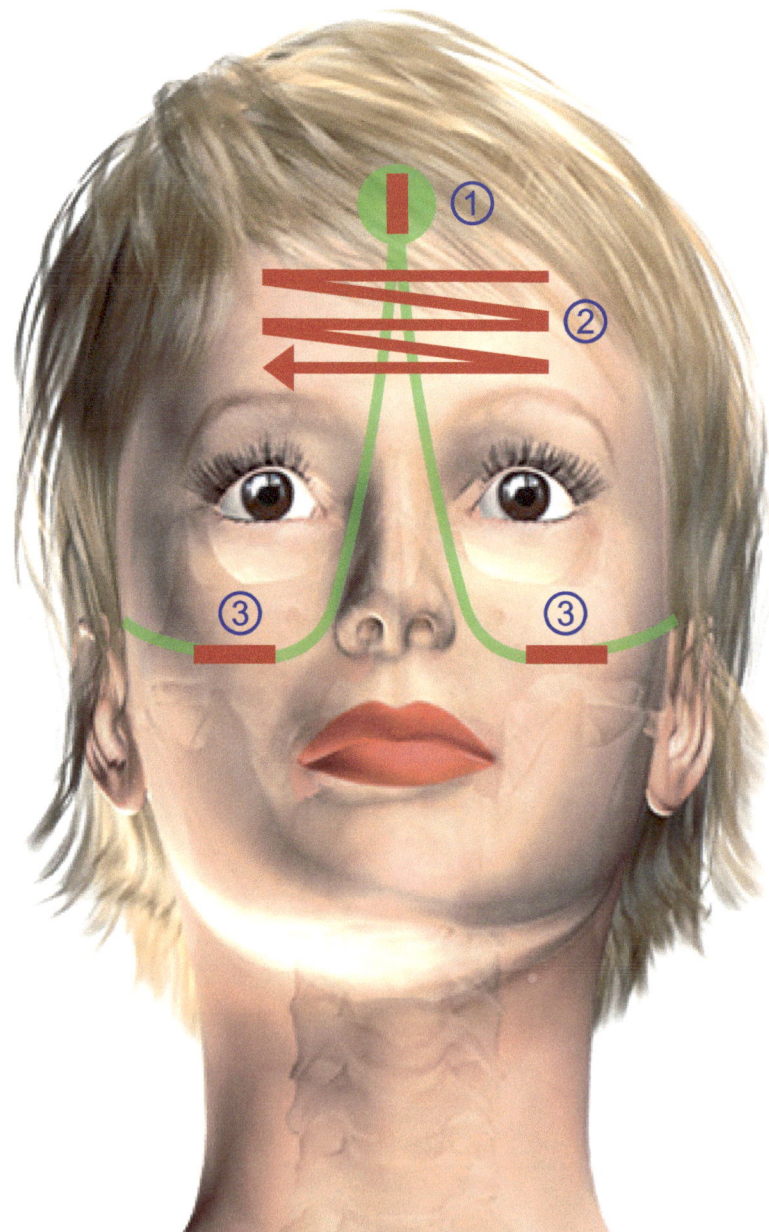

Treatment: STROKES

1. PINCH gently the Blue Point.

2. STROKE the forehead along the Blue Arrows.

3. EXPAND the Blue Points with 2 fingers (reverse movement of pinch)

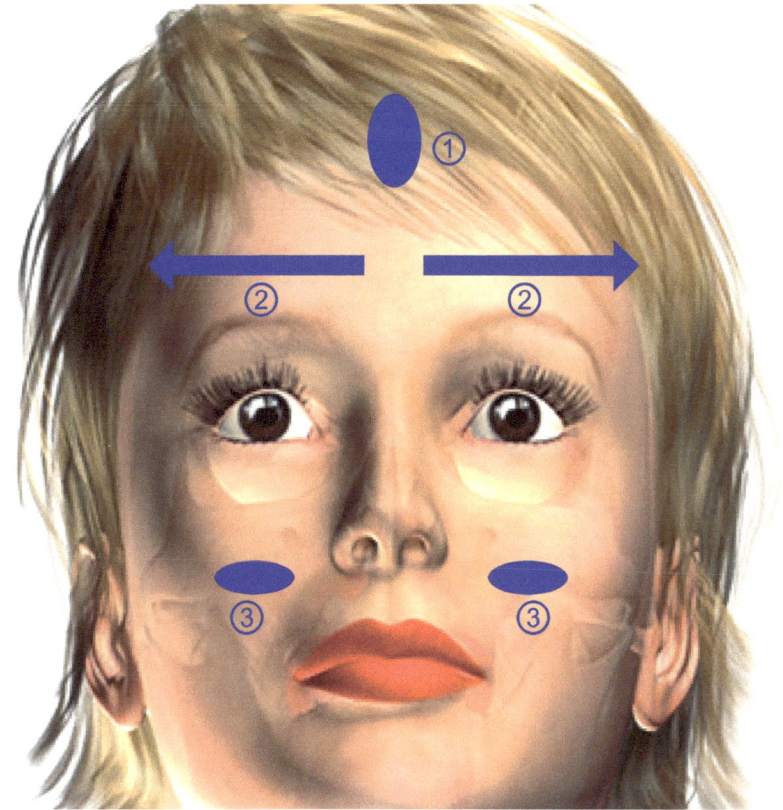

TIP!
Try closing one side of your nostrils with a finger and breath through your nose. You may notice that either side feels slightly stuffy. Everyone has that!

WIDEN THE RESPIRATORY TRACT

Mechanism:

The tension on sternocleidomastoids (side neck muscles) is obviously the most dominant along the neck.
Additionally, myofascial tension between the face and the chest shortens the front of the neck and re-strains the throat.

⚠️ It is important to be very gentle when treating the neck, as it contains extremely delicate arteries and glands such as the thyroid.

Treatment:

1. Gently **STROKE** the neck in the direction of the Blue Arrows along sternocleidomastoids, with the palm of your hands.

2. **SCRATCH** the chin along Red Line to release sticking myofascia from chin-bone edge.

TIP!
Try raising up your chin to feel the tension between the face and the chest.

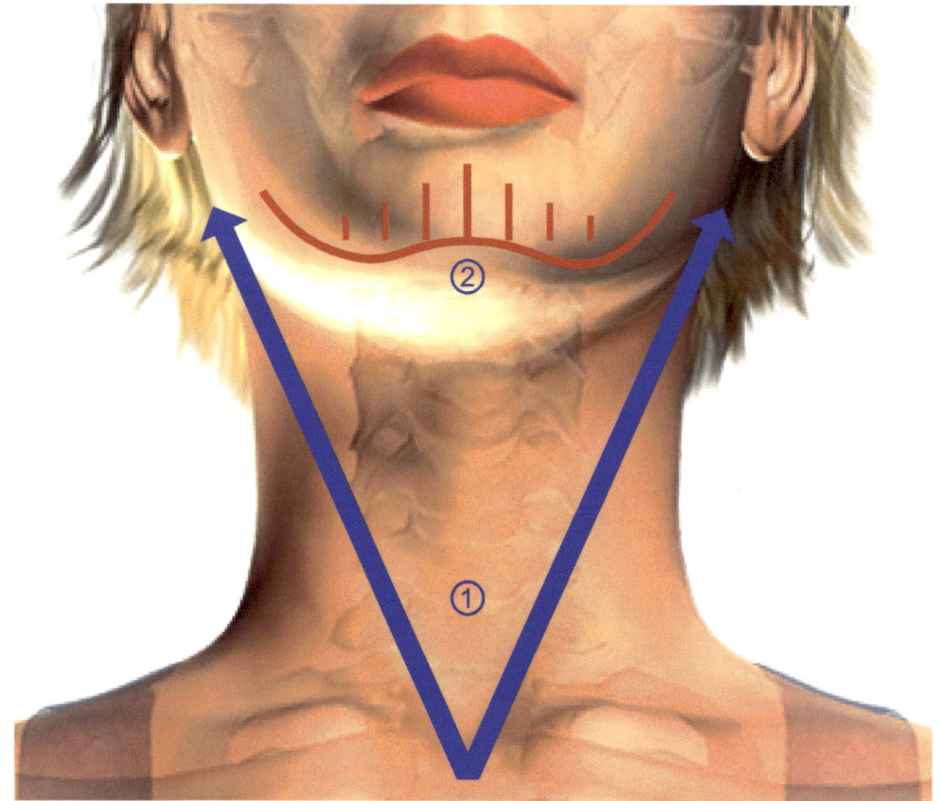

WIDEN THE RIB CAGE

Mechanism:

To breath without restriction, it is important to re-lease any tension around the rib cage. The treatment is divided into 3 regions of the rib cage:

1. The STERNUM: Releasing the tension around the sternum enhances flexibility and increases air vol-ume capacity.

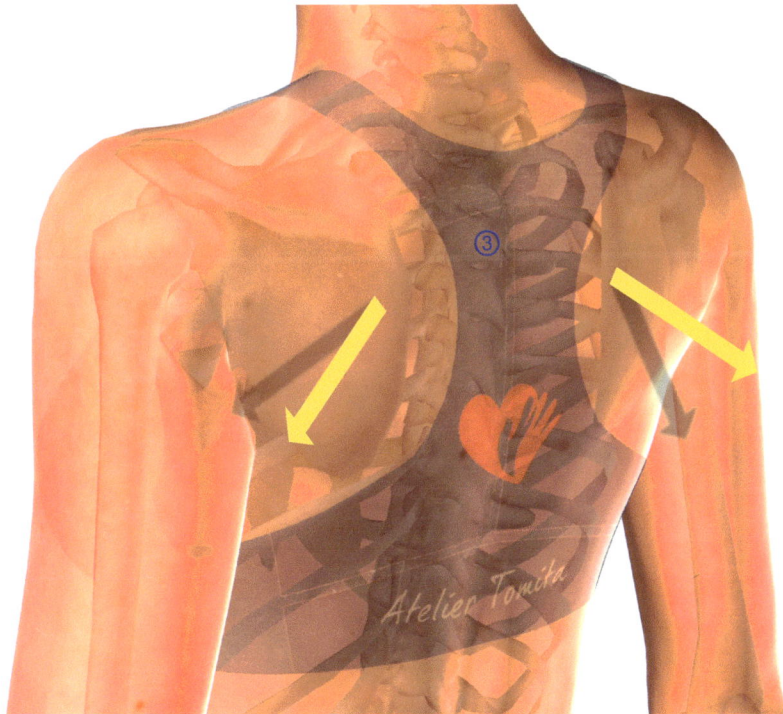

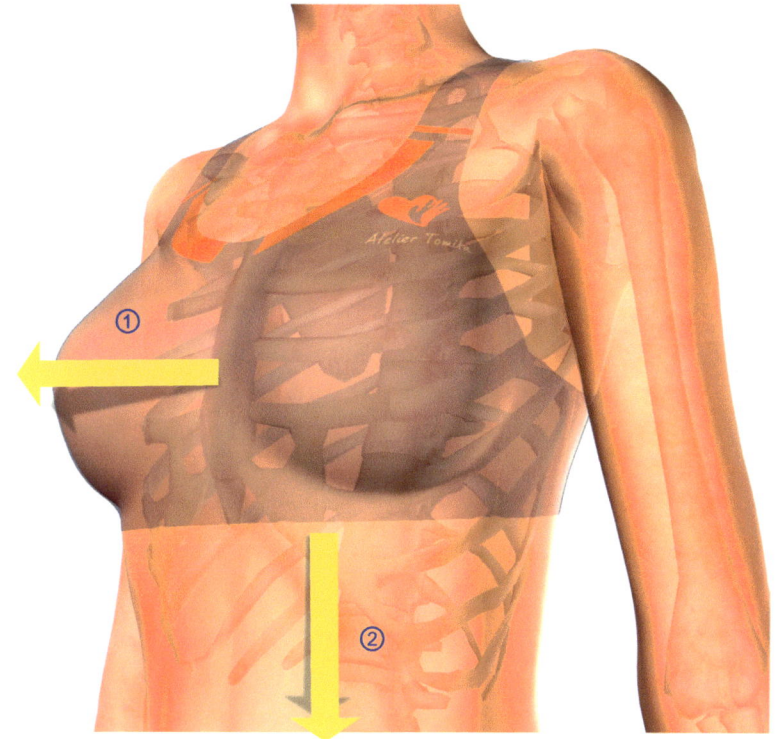

2. The DIAPHRAGM: The tension on the diaphragm comes from the inside part of the rib cage, which is connected by myofascia from the clavicle to the inner thighs. Massaging the rib cage shows to be rather inefficient. It is thus better to work on the inner thighs' tension to soften the diaphragm.

3. The UPPER BACK: Smoothness of the upper back of the body is a major factor to improve breath-ing. This rather complex area is treated in part from the back of the head.

1 STERNUM

Treatment: SCRATCHING

1. SCRATCH the Red Lines and SLIDE to the side (Meridian Point CV17)

2. SCRATCH the joints between sternum and rib cage, and SLIDE a little outward laterally

3. SCRATCH right below the clavicles and SLIDE outward laterally

4. SCRATCH right below the humerus and SLIDE downward medially

⚠️ This usually hurts a lot when performed for the first time. It is important to start gently and reassure the patient that this pain will quickly fade away and will not come back if self-treated regularly.

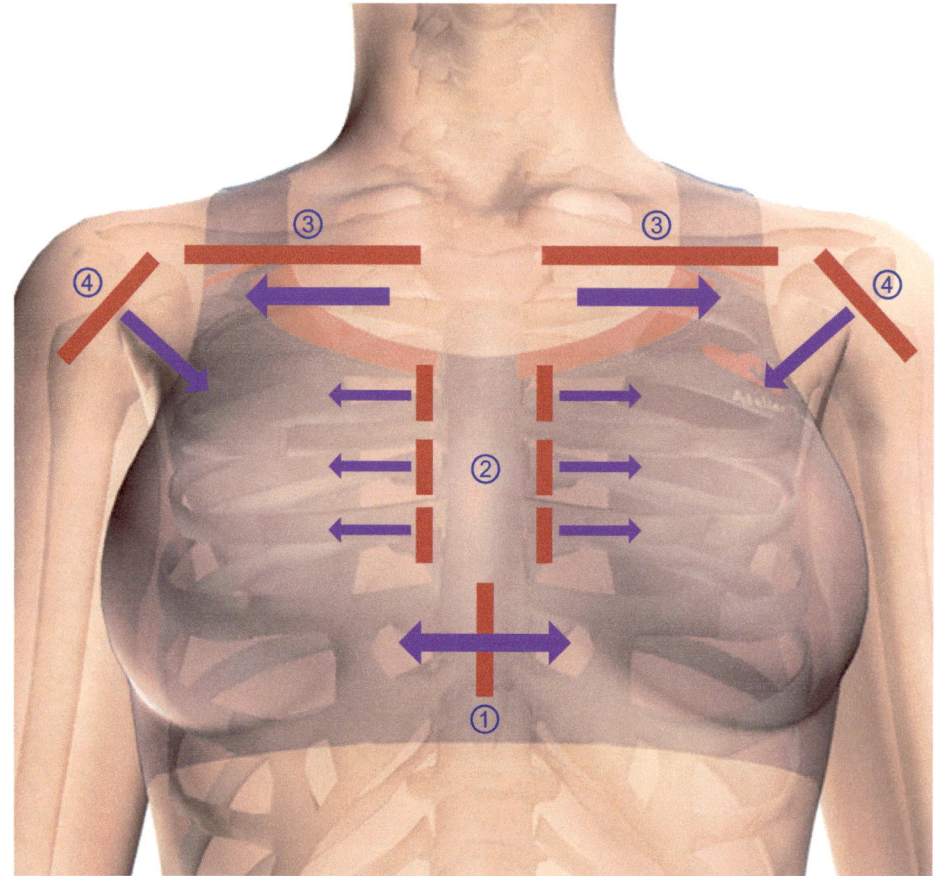

Treatment: STROKES

When the patient's sternum is too painful, it is better to use the GENTLE STROKE approach. This method should also be taught to the patient for self-care maintenance.

1. STROKE the sternum upward.

2. STROKE the rib cage to lateral

3. STROKE the clavicles to medial

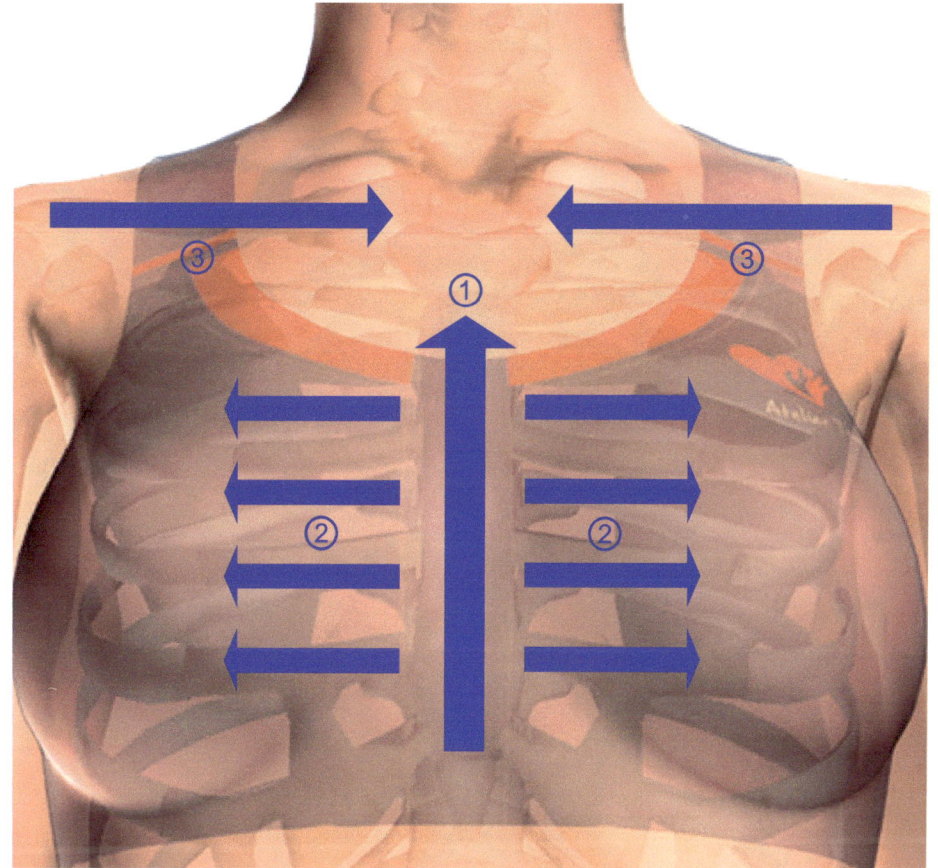

TIP!
The greater tuberosity of humerus usually naturally touches down the massage bed after performing this treatment, when the patient lays face up.

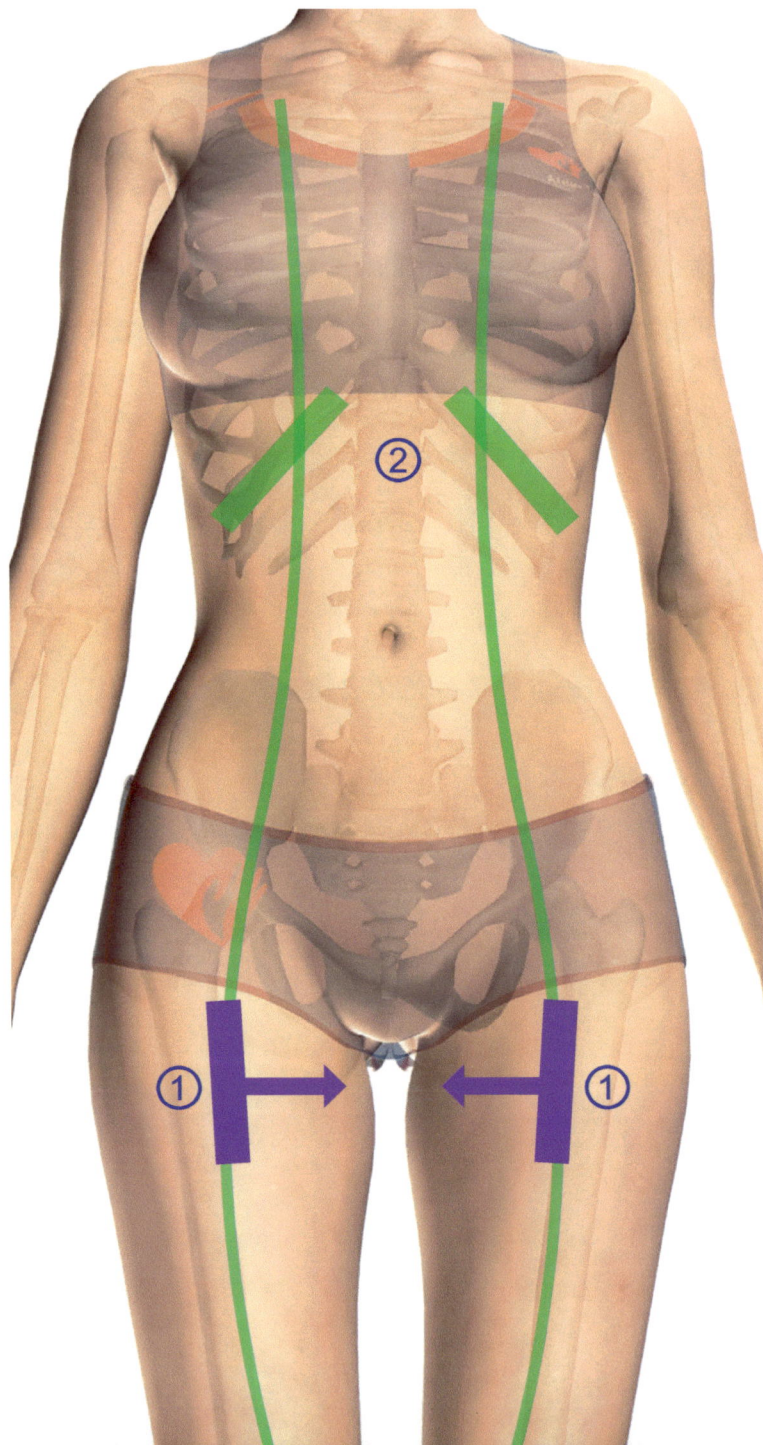

2 DIAPHRAGM

Mechanism:

The stiffness of the diaphragm can be evaluated with the tips of your fingers diagonally down the edge of the rib cage.
The tension is extended along the Green Lines inside the body and causes tension in the inner thighs.

Treatment: SLIDING

1. SLIDE the thigh medial muscle with the Venus hill of your hand as the Purple Arrows show.

2. Verify the diaphragm stiffness as you repeat the treatment on both thighs.

3 UPPER BACK

Mechanism:

Multiple muscles, such as the Erector Spinae and the trapezoid, are attached at one end on the edge of the back head bone. This creates a strong myofascial tension on the back of the head. By releasing this tension, it gives room to the upper back muscles to expand the rib cage more widely.

Treatment: SCRATCHING

1. Search around the Red Areas for hollow spots on the head bone.
1. SCRATCH vigorously around these two Red Areas with your finger nails

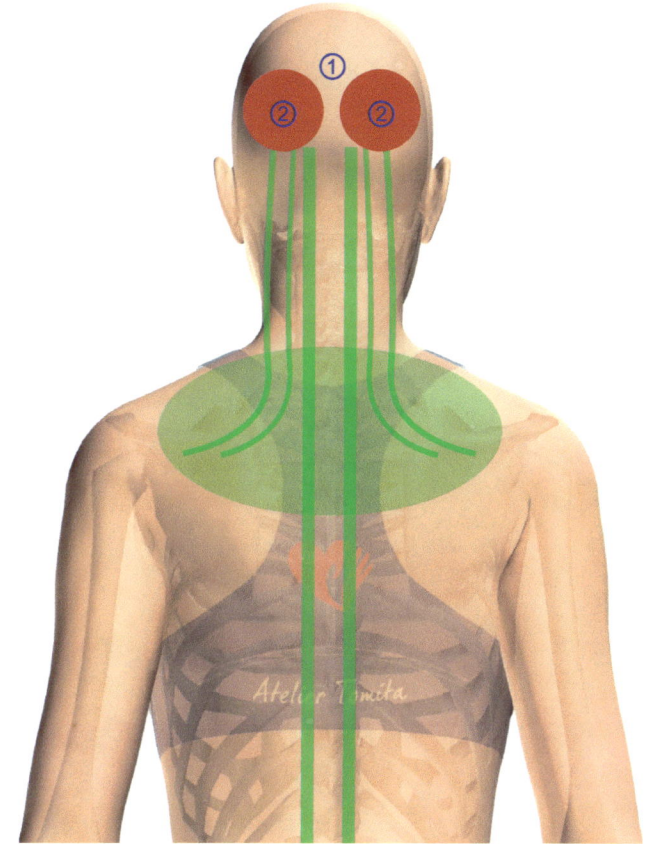

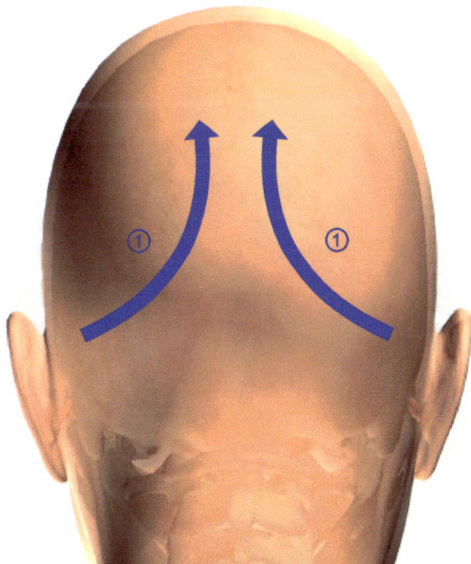

Treatment: STROKES

1. Gently STROKE along the vBlue Arrows with your fingertips

This method can be taught to the patient for self care maintenance.

TIP!
Once the back head tension decreases, you can move your eyebrow smoothly. This method is also very effective for migraines !

EVALUATION

1. How do you widen the nasal cavity?

2. How do you widen the respiratory tract?

3. What are the 3 body parts that you should treat to widen the rib cage?

4. Can you perform the hand techniques?

5. Can you teach some self-care techniques?

NOTES

NECK AND SHOULDERS

OUTLINE

1. Understanding neck and shoulder pain
2. Releasing tension on fingers and palm
3. Releasing tension on the forearm
4. Releasing tension on the upper arm

UNDERSTANDING NECK AND SHOULDER PAIN

Mechanism:

The neck and shoulders are mid way of the myofascial connection between the hands and head. It is a very complex area, comprising several specific connection lines along the arms. The basic approach to release pain an tension on the neck and shoulder area is to take care of the hands and arms, which are at one end of the connection lines.

There are two principal lines:
1. The Posterior Hand Index Lateral Line
2. The Posterior Hand Little Finger Medial Line

Identify first which part of the shoulder and neck is mostly affected and apply the proper treatments along the corresponding line.

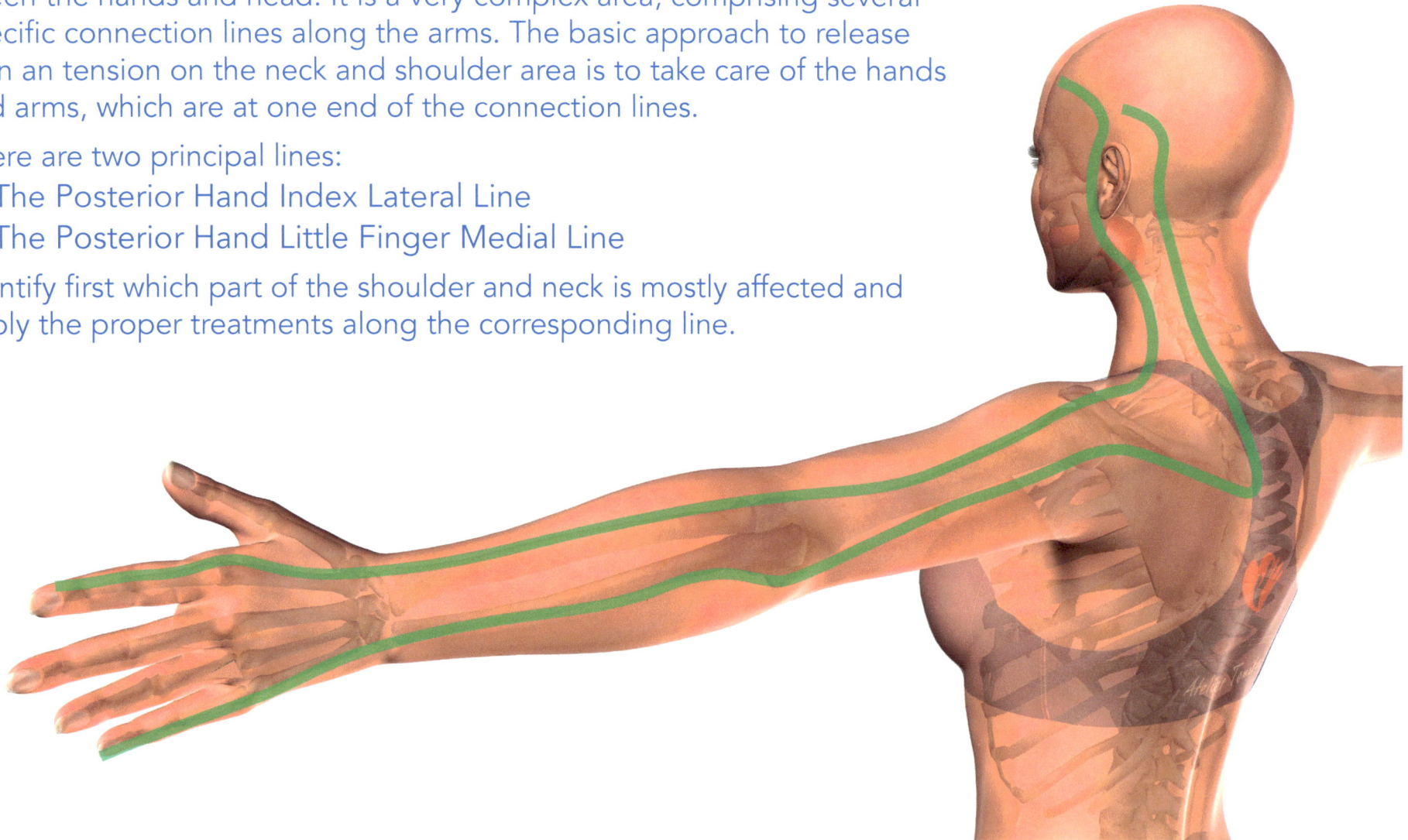

POSTERIOR HAND INDEX LATERAL LINE

As shown on the pictures, myofascial tension stretches along the Green Line, from the frontal top of the head, through the side of the neck, on the top of the shoulder and along the arm, to finish in the index. The treatment points are on the bone edges marked by Red Lines.

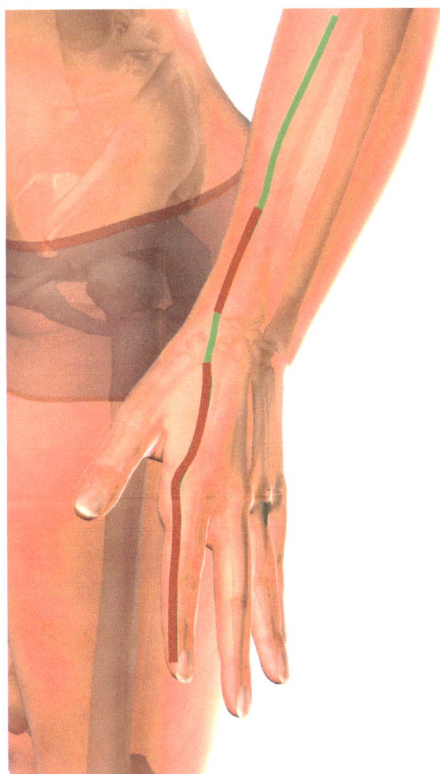

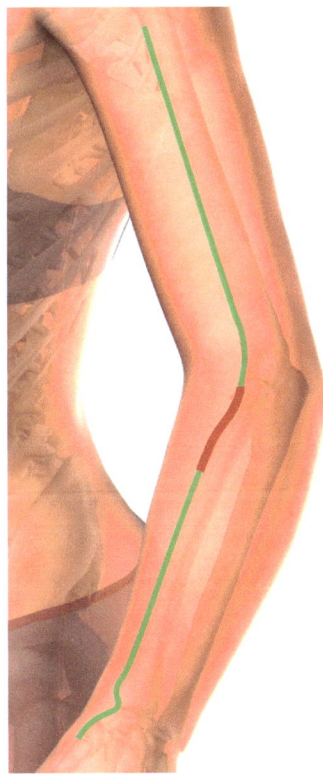

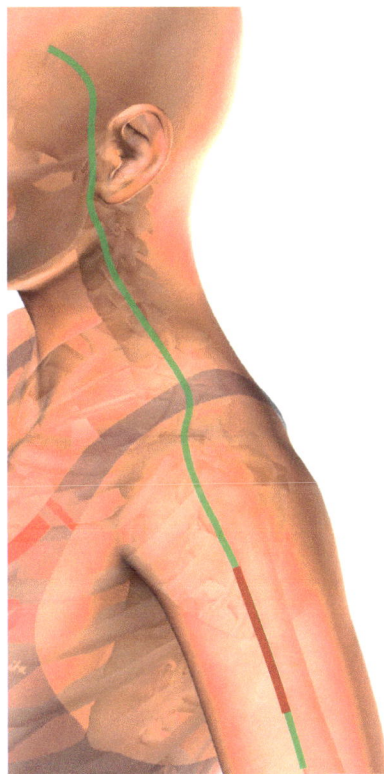

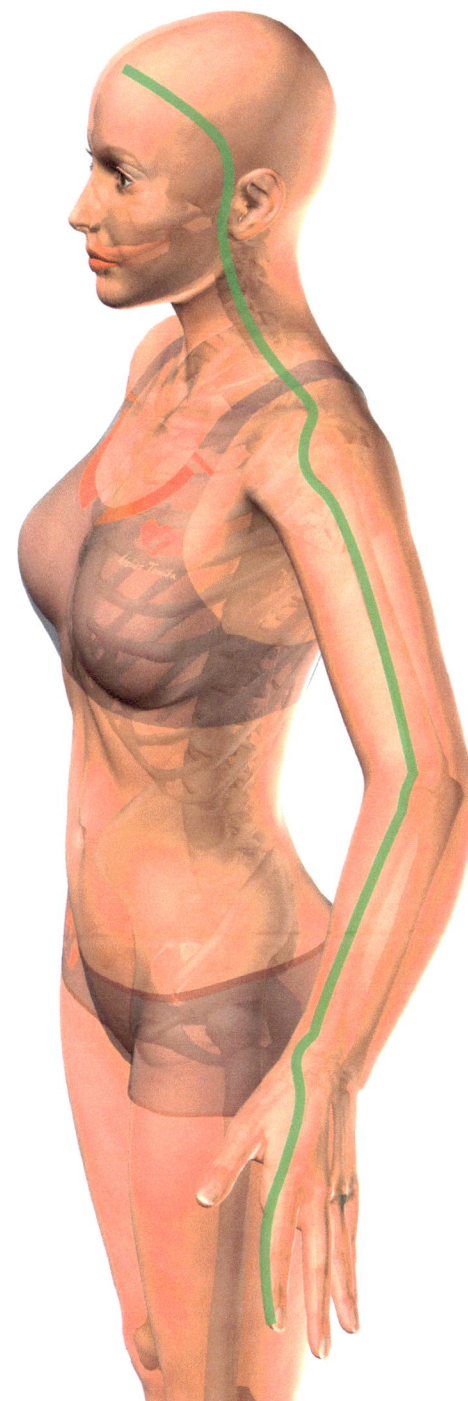

See also:
Superficial Back Arm Line - Anatomy Train
Yangming of hand meridian muscle - Jing jin

POSTERIOR HAND LITTLE FINGER MEDIAL LINE

Myofascial tension also stretches from above the ear, through the back of the neck, around the Scapula and through the shoulder, down along the back of the arm to end in the side of the little finger. It is shown with the Green Line on the picture, and the treatment points are located on the bone edges marked by Red Lines

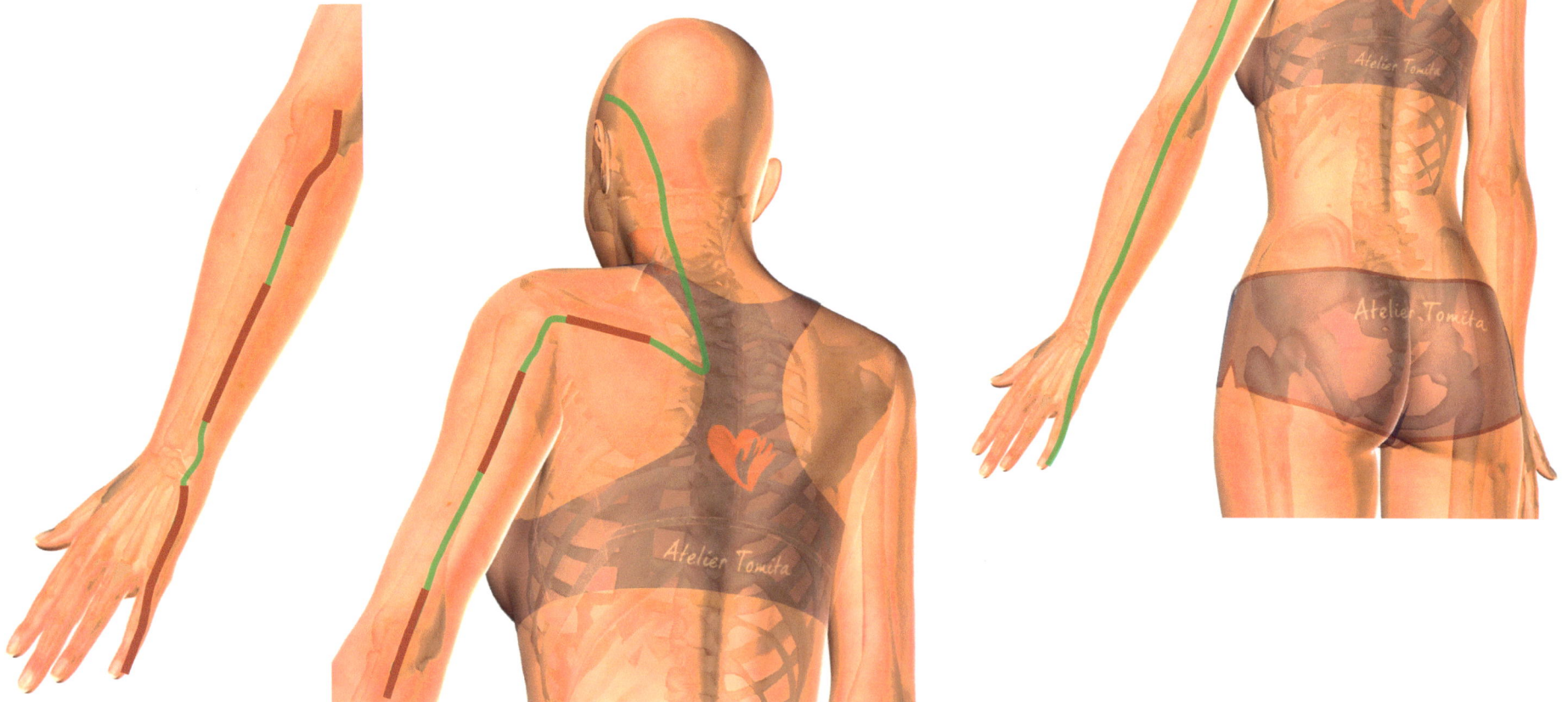

See also:
Deep Back Arm Line - Anatomy Train
Taiyang of hand meridian muscle - Jing jin

RELEASING TENSION ON FINGERS AND PALM

To release tension of the neck and shoulder, start with the fingers and palms. This time we will focus on the index and the little fingers, but the hand techniques will apply to other fingers further in the course. You will use both SCRATCHING and STROKES.

Treatment 1: SCRATCHING

1. SCRATCH the proximal edge of each Phalanges (slightly toward the anterior edge)
2. SCRATCH the proximal edge of each Phalanges (slightly toward the posterior edge)
3. SCRATCH between metacarpals

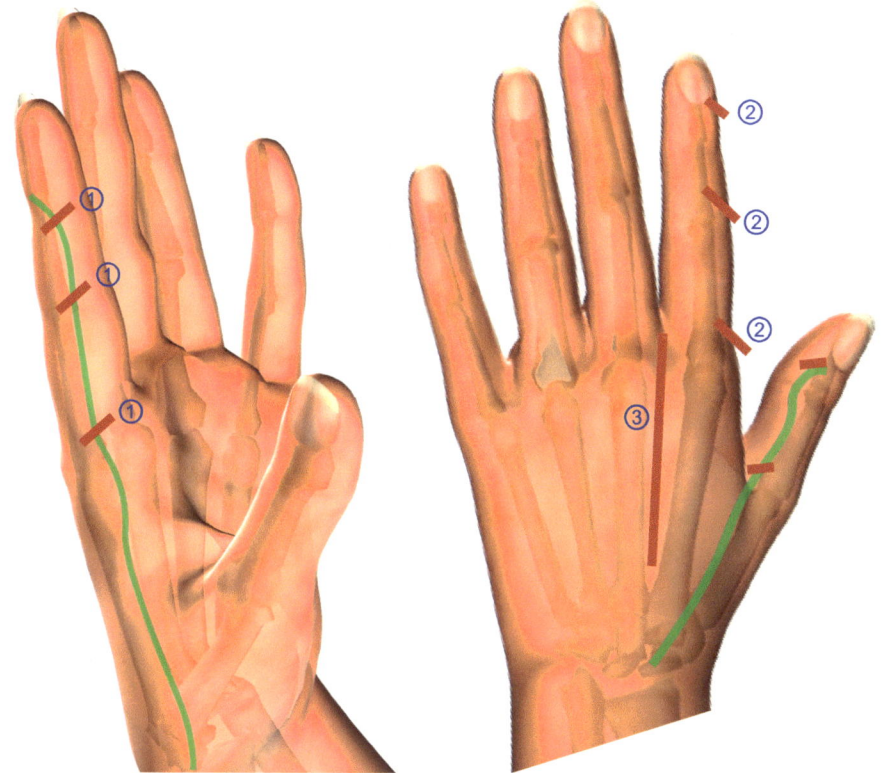

TIP!

These images mainly show how to release tension on posterior hand index lateral line. The thumb medial edge also connects with this line. Each finger has 2 myofascial lines on both (medial/lateral) sides. Try to twist the finger gently, and if it's too hard to twist, release the tension with this technique.

Treatment 2: SCRATCHING

1. SCRATCH the proximal edge of each Phalanges
   (slightly toward the anterior edge)
   (slightly toward the posterior edge)

2. SCRATCH the proximal edge of the Metacarpal
   and SLIDE it to anterior

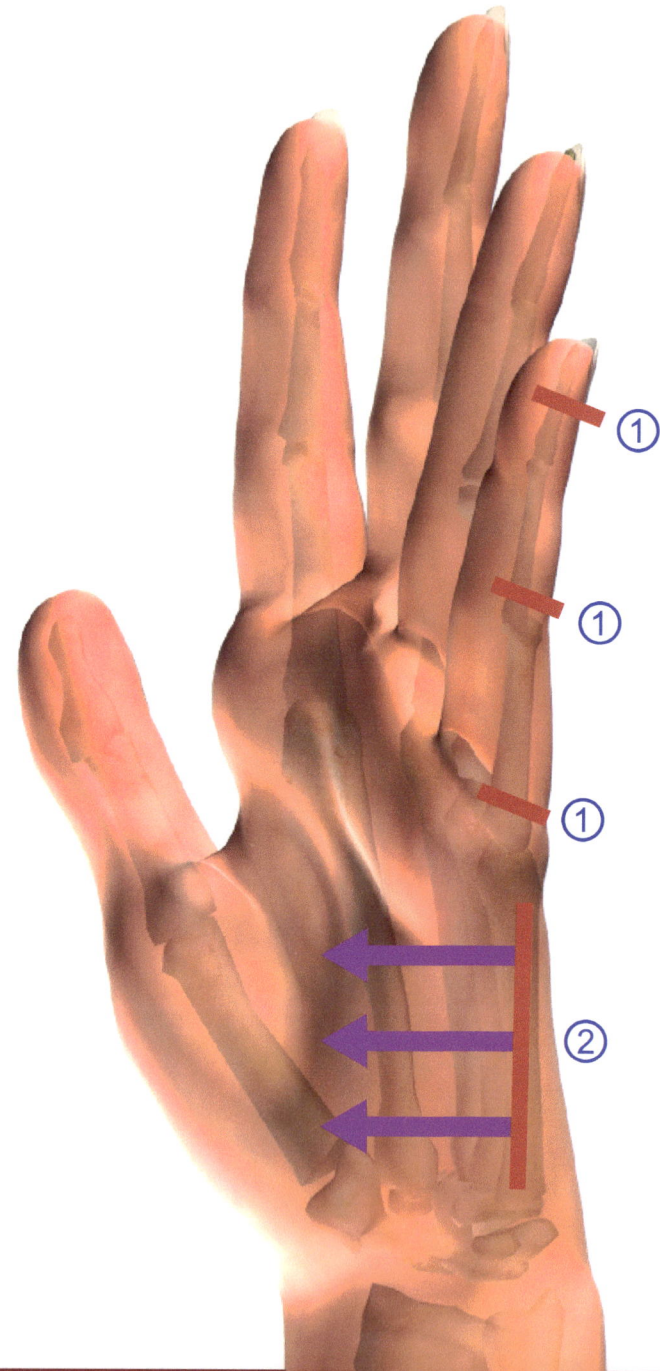

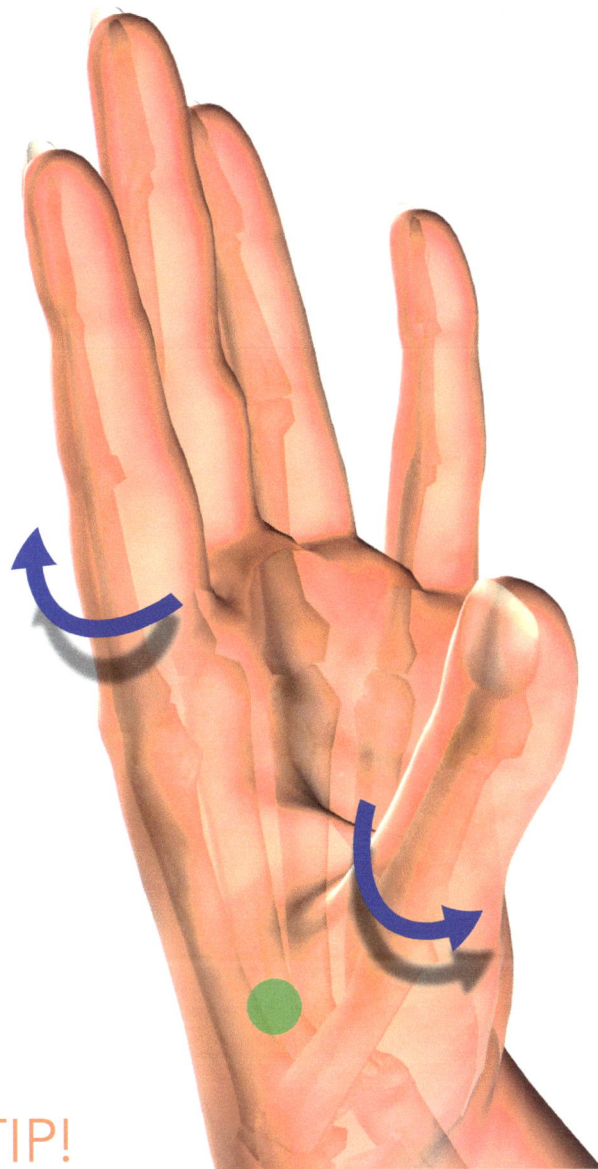

Treatment 3: STROKES

1. STROKE the index like wounding from proximal to distal

2. STROKE the thumb like wounding from proximal to distal

3. Check the stiffness at green point (Meridian Point LI4)

This technique is very gentle and very easy and can be taught to your patient for self-care maintenance.

TIP!

The thumb oppose the rest of the fingers in the hand's natural position. But with computer work, the part at the green point narrows and stiffens, which opens and flattens the hand. These STROKES release the tensions on the fingers, and bring them back to their natural position.

RELEASING TENSION ON FOREARM

Treatment: SCRATCHING

1. SCRATCH the distal edge of the Radius and SLIDE it to medial
2. SCRATCH the proximal edge of the Radius and SLIDE it to medial
3. SCRATCH the distal edge of the Ulna and SLIDE it to lateral

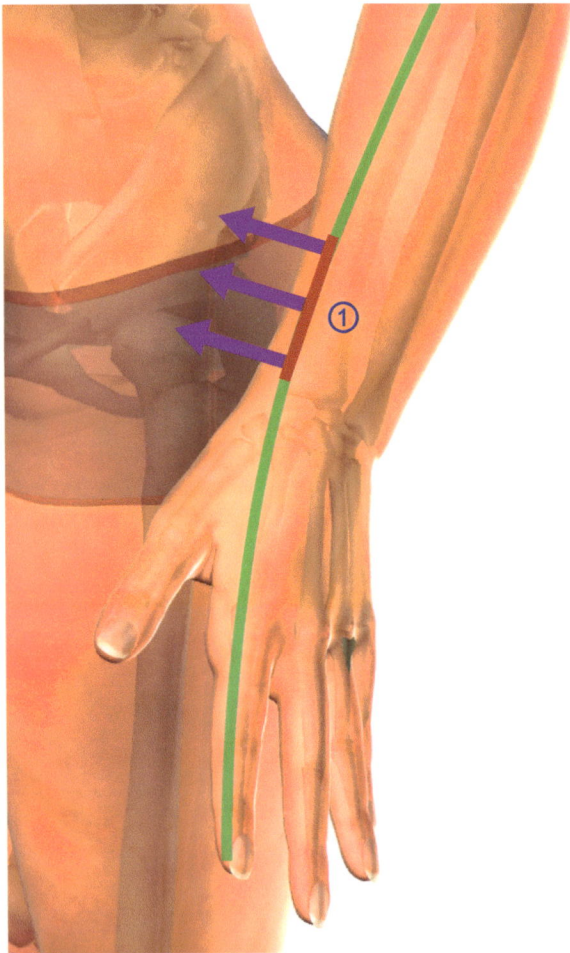

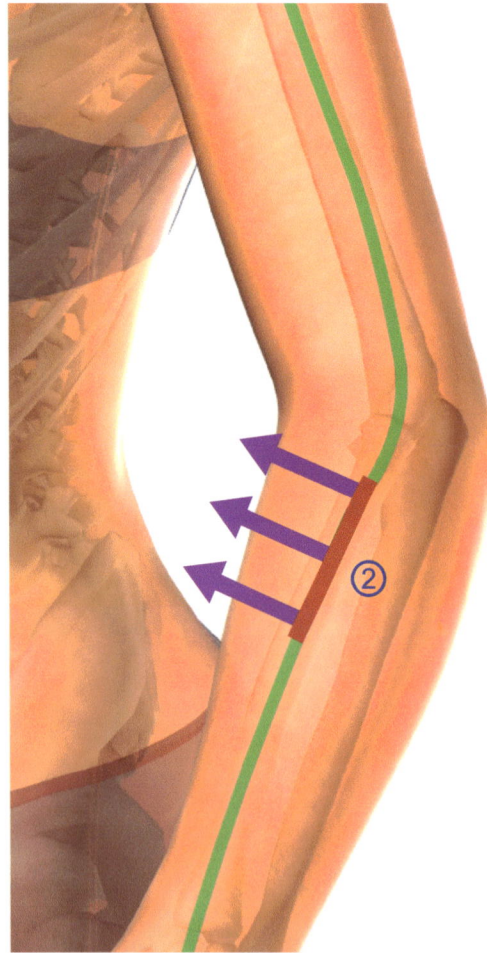

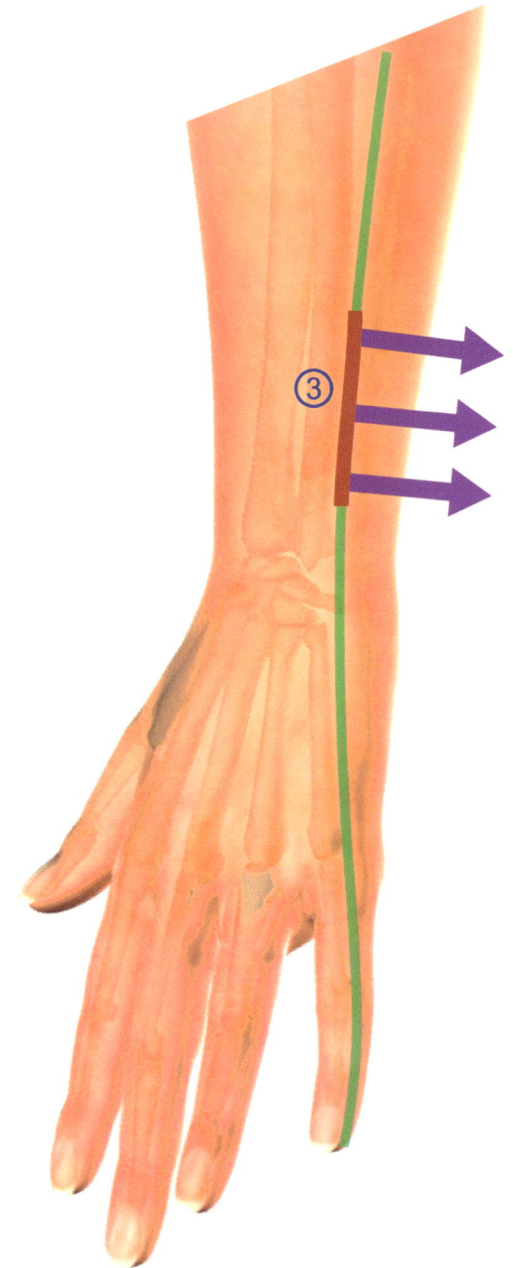

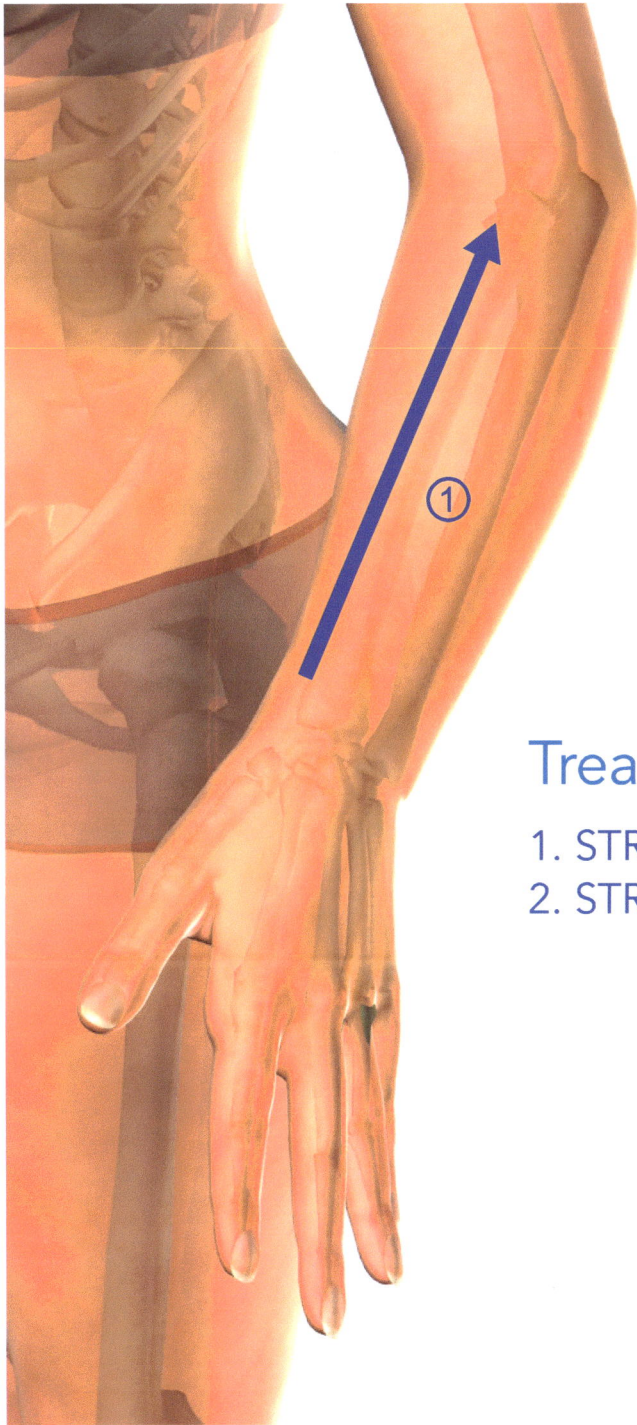

You can use gentle strokes as well. They can be easily performed as self-care by your patient, whenever they feel some stiffness in their shoulder and neck.

Treatment: STROKES

1. STROKE along the Radius from distal to proximal
2. STROKE along the Ulna from proximal to distal

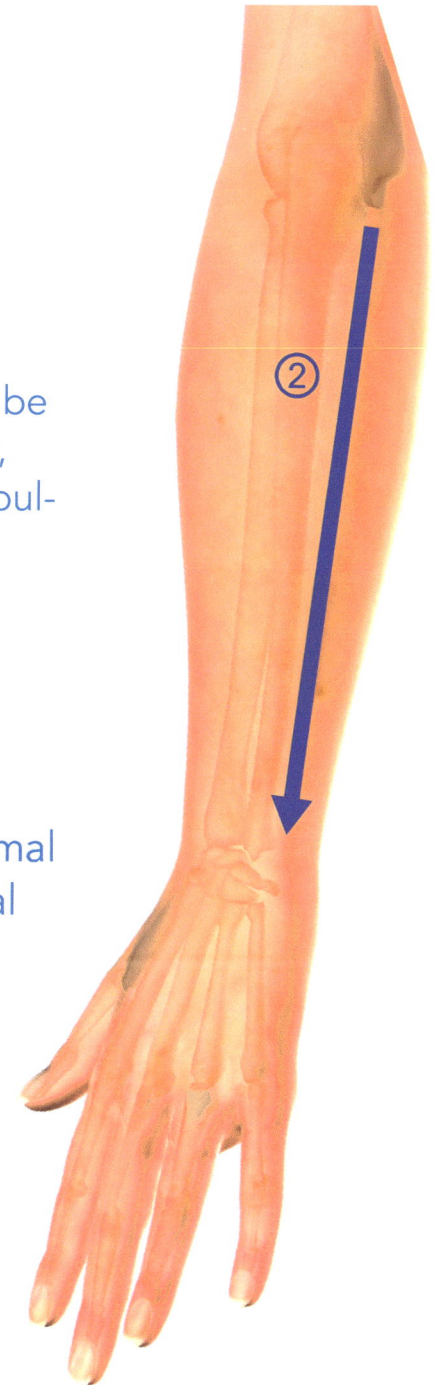

RELEASING TENSION ON UPPER ARM

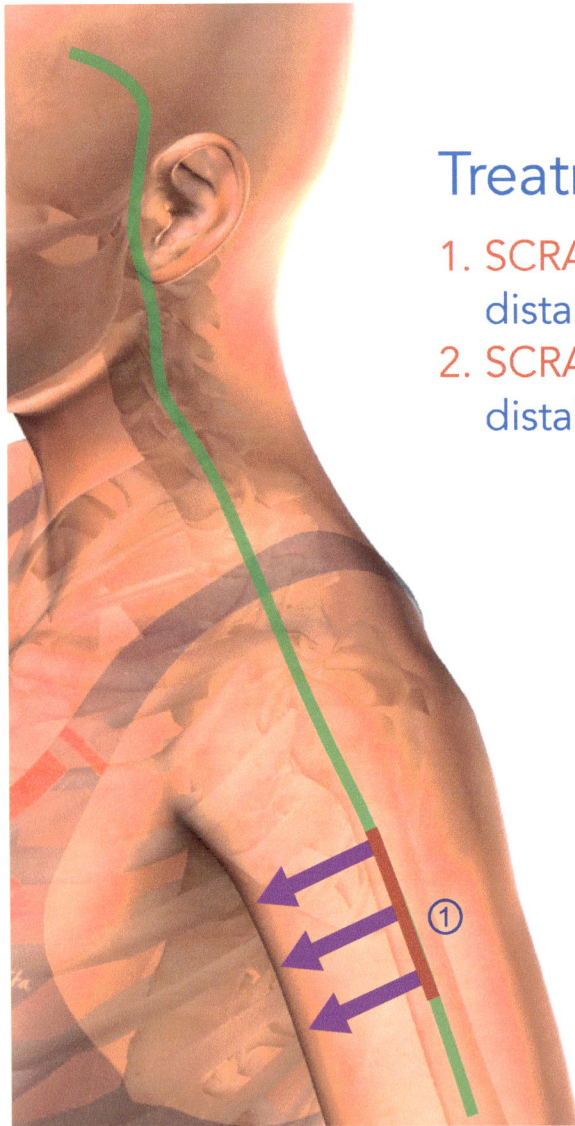

Treatment: SCRATCHING

1. SCRATCH the proximal edge of the Humerus (around the distal edge of the Deltoid) and SLIDE it to medial
2. SCRATCH the proximal edge of the Humerus (around the distal edge of Deltoid) and SLIDE it to medial

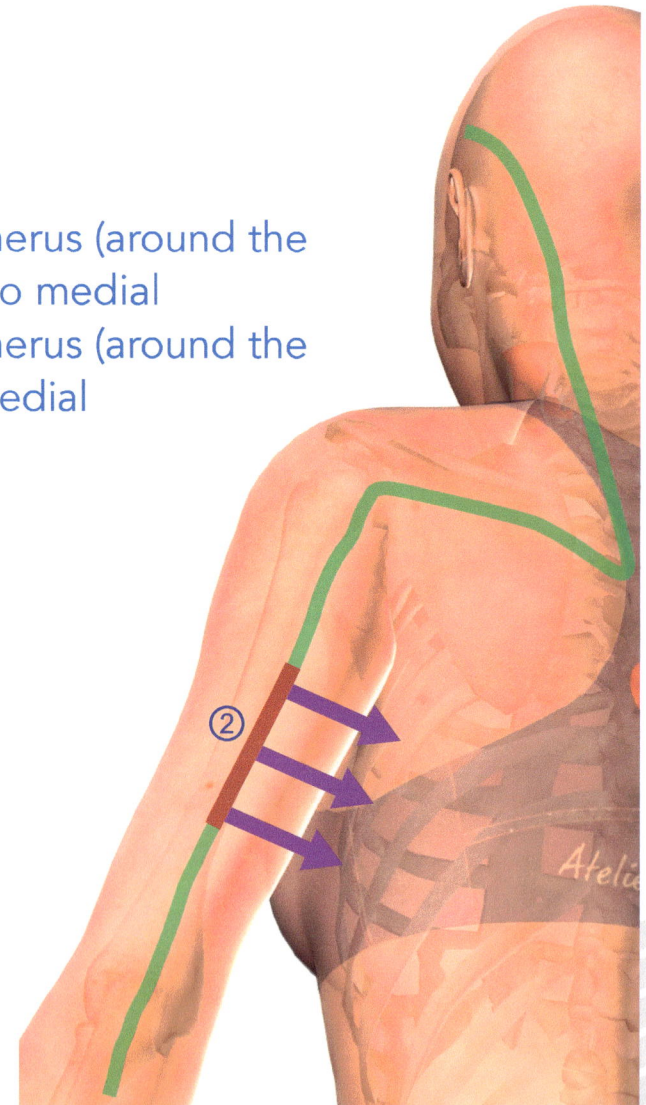

Treatment: STROKES

1. STROKE along the Humerus from proximal to distal

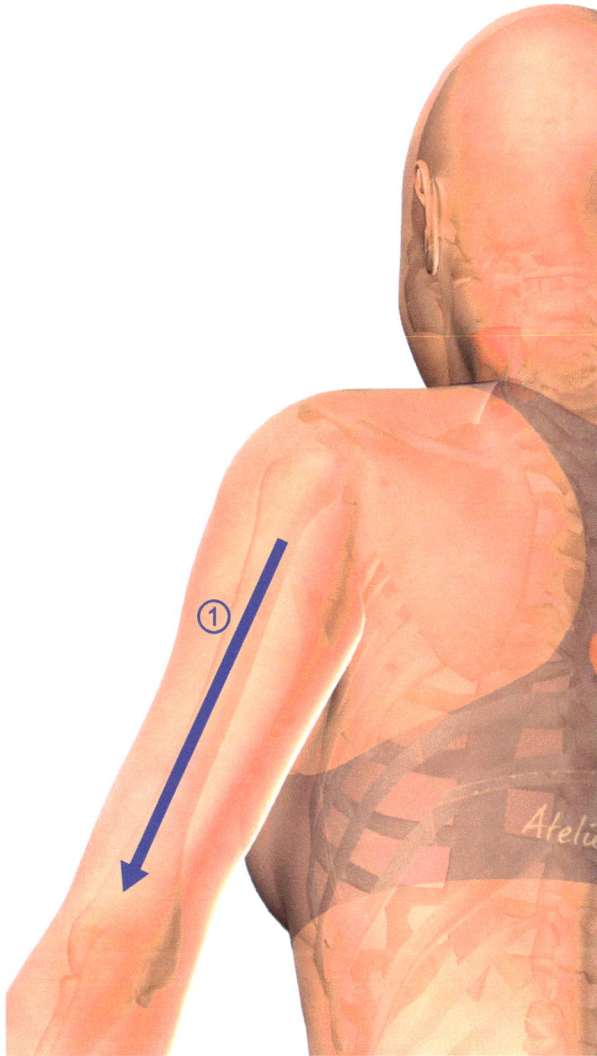

This method is very effective and also easy to perform as self-care by the patient.

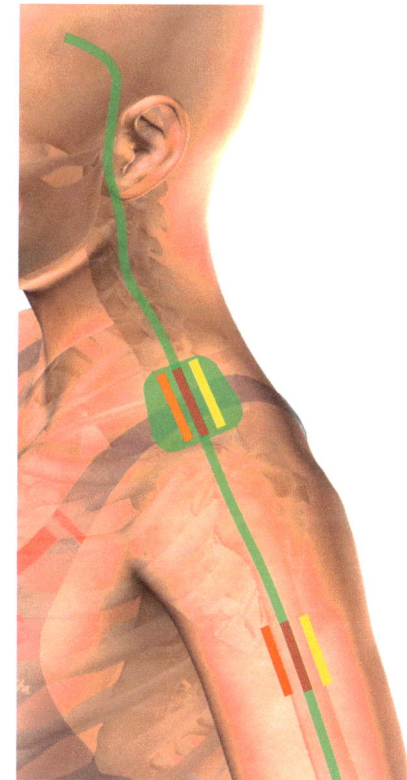

TIP !
To release pain at the base of the neck (green square), focus on the stiff points on the side of the shoulder, according to its connecting line (see image above).

EVALUATION

1. Can you identify the two main myofascial tension lines along the neck and shoulders?

2. Can you release the tension on the finger and palms?

3. Can you release the tension on the forearm?

4. Can you release the tension on the upper arm?

5. What self-care methods would you teach your patient?

NOTES

ARM AND FROZEN SHOULDER

OUTLINE

1. Understanding arm and frozen shoulder pain
2. Releasing tension on fingers
3. Releasing tension on the elbow
4. Releasing tension under the armpit
5. Understanding our unconscious posture and how it is linked to arm pain
6. Effective ways to use our arms

UNDERSTANDING ARM AND FROZEN SHOULDER PAIN

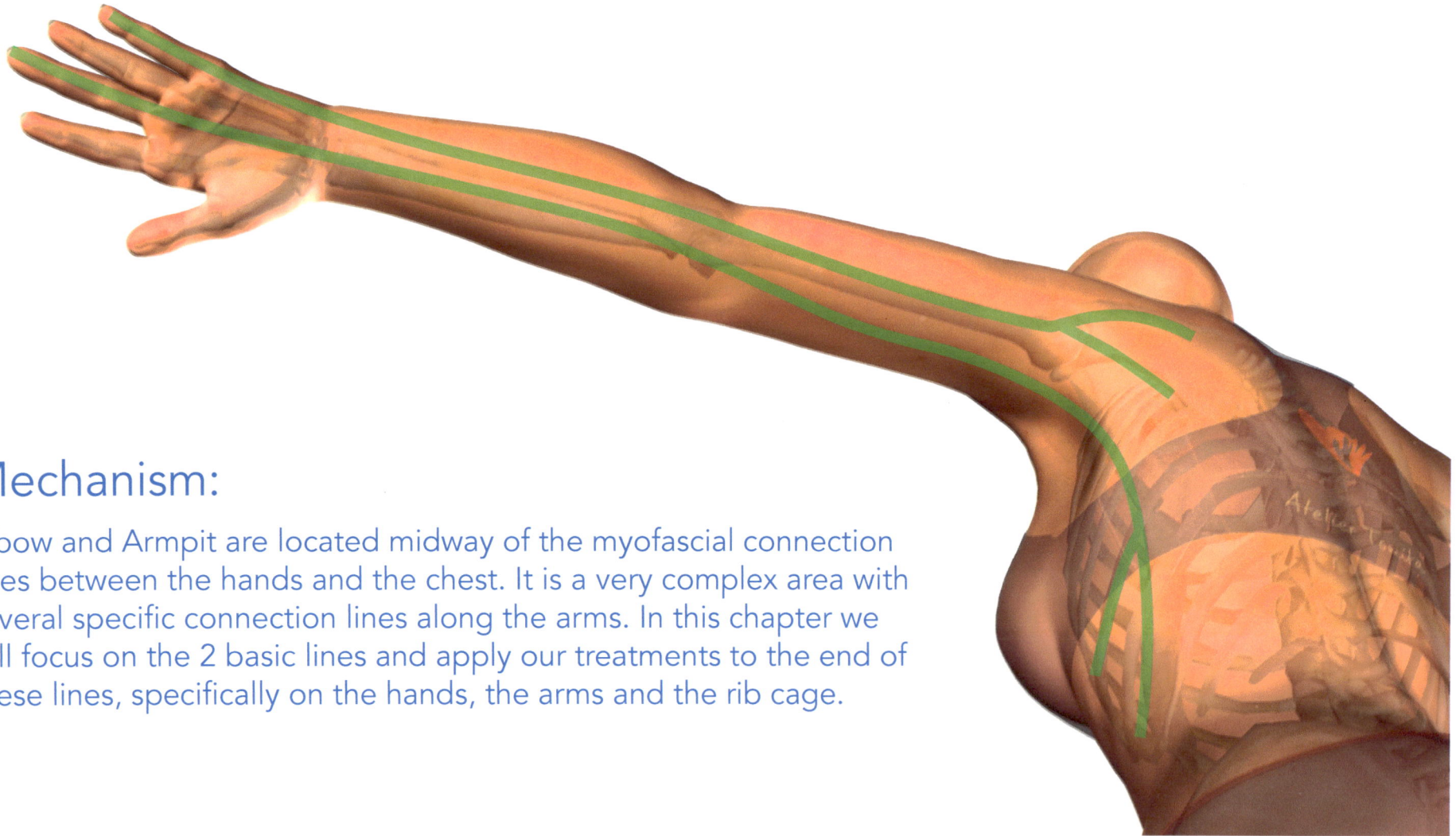

Mechanism:

Elbow and Armpit are located midway of the myofascial connection lines between the hands and the chest. It is a very complex area with several specific connection lines along the arms. In this chapter we will focus on the 2 basic lines and apply our treatments to the end of these lines, specifically on the hands, the arms and the rib cage.

ANTERIOR HAND LITTLE FINGER MEDIAL LINE

Myofascial tension shown along the Green Line stretches from the Scapula to the tip of the little finger. The treatment points are located on the bone edges marked in red.

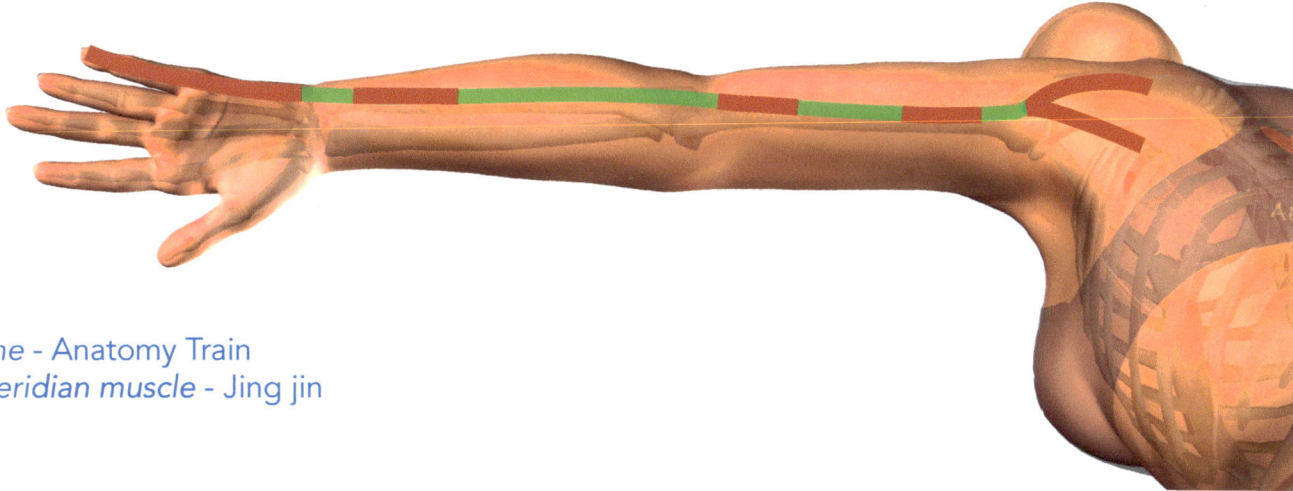

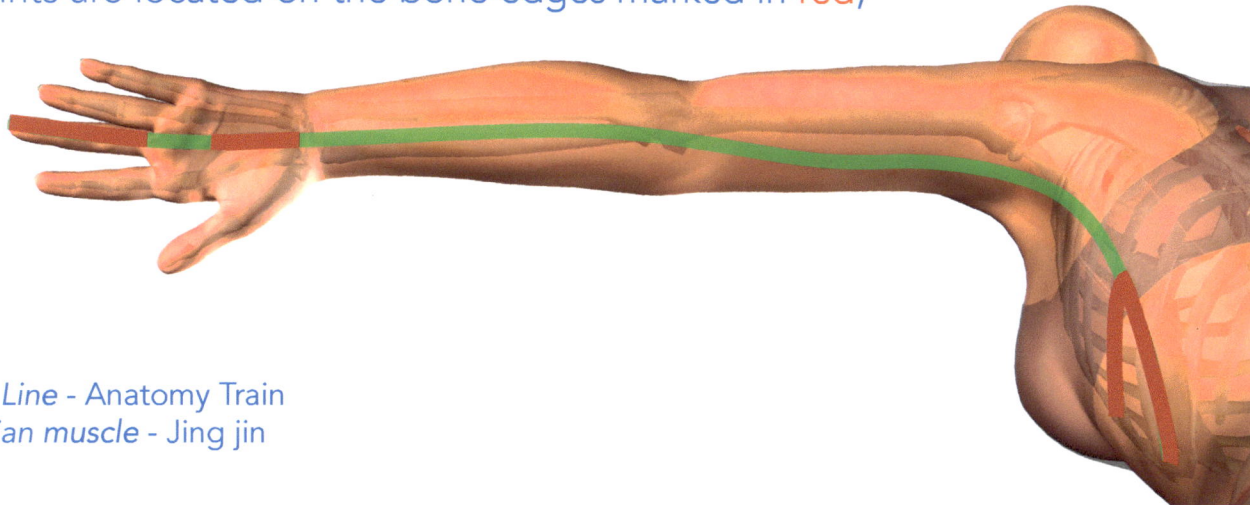

See also:
Deep Back Arm Line - Anatomy Train
Taiyang of hand meridian muscle - Jing jin

ANTERIOR HAND MIDDLE FINGER MEDIAL LINE

Myofascial tension shown along the Green Line stretches from the rib cage to the tip of the middle finger. The treatment points are located on the bone edges marked in red,

See also:
Superficial Front Arm Line - Anatomy Train
JueYin of hand meridian muscle - Jing jin

RELEASING TENSION ON FINGERS

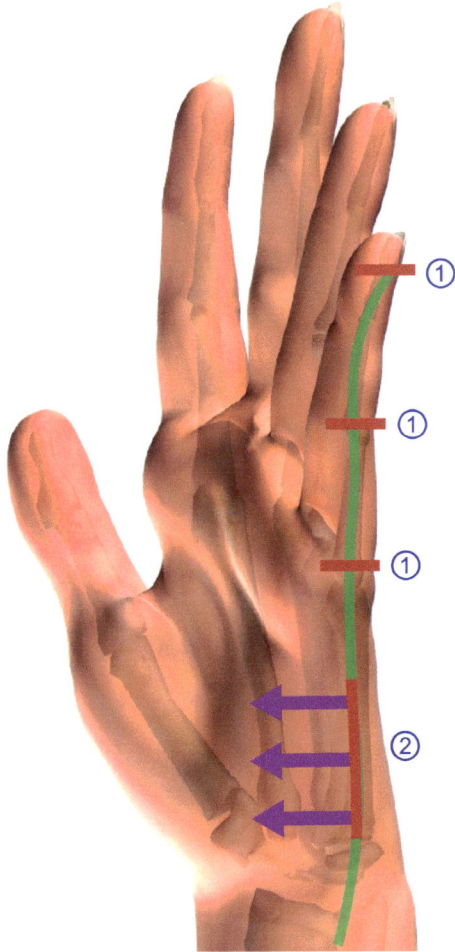

Treatment: SCRATCHES

1. **SCRATCH** the proximal edge of each Phalanges
   (a little toward the anterior edge)
   (a little toward the posterior edge)

2. **SCRATCH** the proximal edge of Metacarpal and **SLIDE** it to anterior

3. **SCRATCH** the proximal edge of each Phalanges
   (a little toward the anterior edge)
   (a little toward the posterior edge)

4. **SCRATCH** between Metacarpals

5. **SCRATCH** around the Capitate and **SLIDE** it to the side

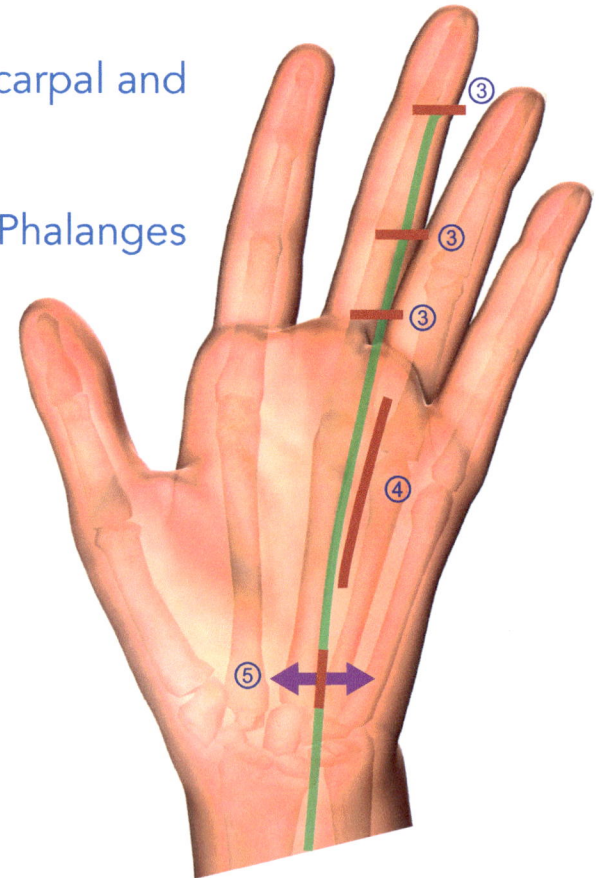

TIP!
Try to twist fingers gently to check the stiffness. Once the tension decreases, they may be easier to twist.

RELEASING TENSION ON ELBOW

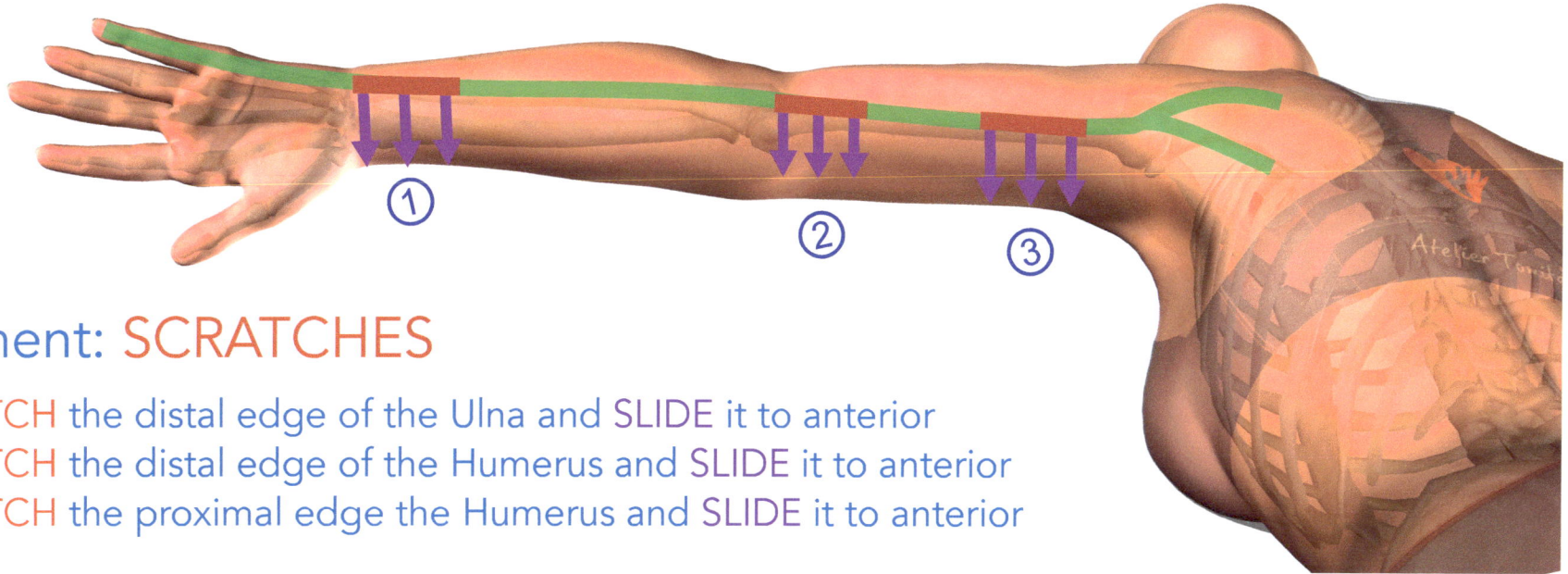

Treatment: SCRATCHES

1. SCRATCH the distal edge of the Ulna and SLIDE it to anterior
2. SCRATCH the distal edge of the Humerus and SLIDE it to anterior
3. SCRATCH the proximal edge the Humerus and SLIDE it to anterior

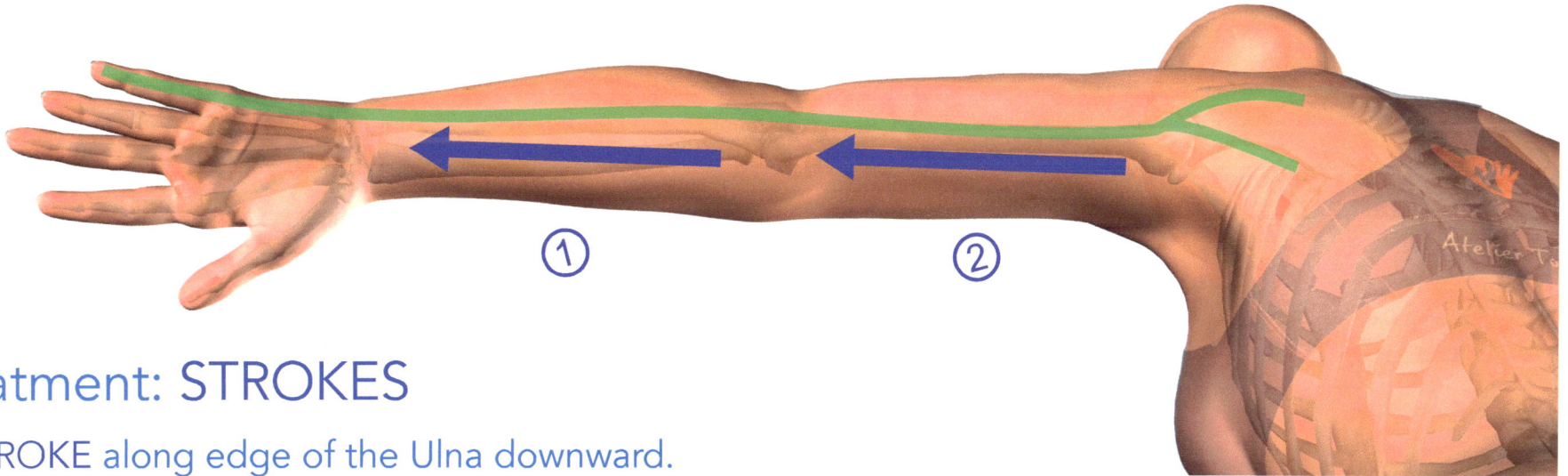

Treatment: STROKES

1. STROKE along edge of the Ulna downward.
2. STROKE along edge of the Humerus downward.

RELEASING TENSION UNDER THE ARMPIT

Treatment: SCRATCHES

1. SCRATCH the Axillary border of the Scapula and SLIDE it to anterior (the edge is the anterior side of the Scapula)
2. SCRATCH beneath the spine of the Scapula and SLIDE it to inferior (the edge is the posterior side of the Scapula)
3. SCRATCH the edge of the rib cage

⚠️ The armpit is a very delicate part of the body, it is a passage for a lot of nerves and veins, which is not protected by muscles. It is a very sensitive area. Tell the patient first that you will be touching the armpit, then gently feel the shape of the bones before your start treating.

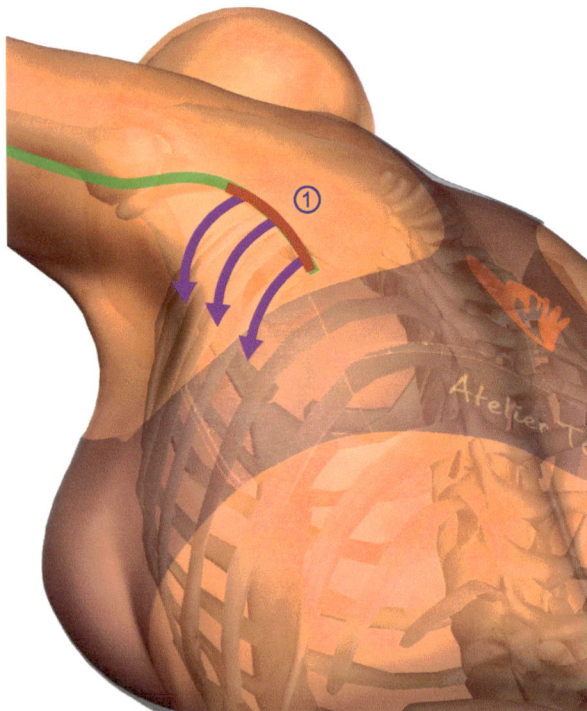

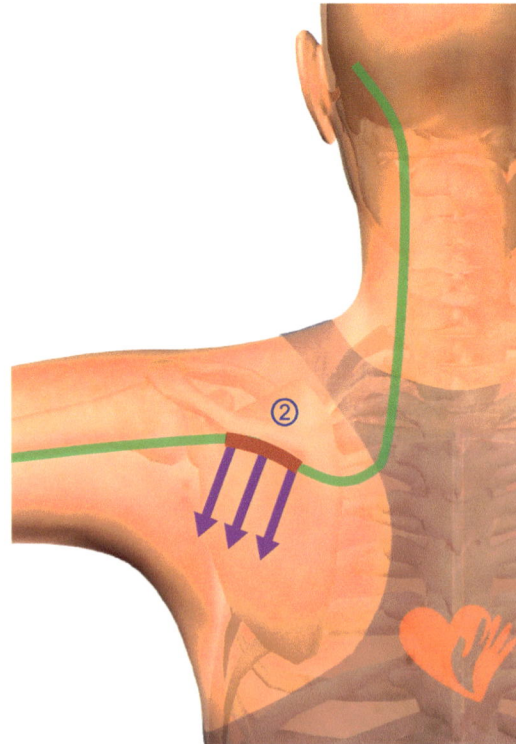

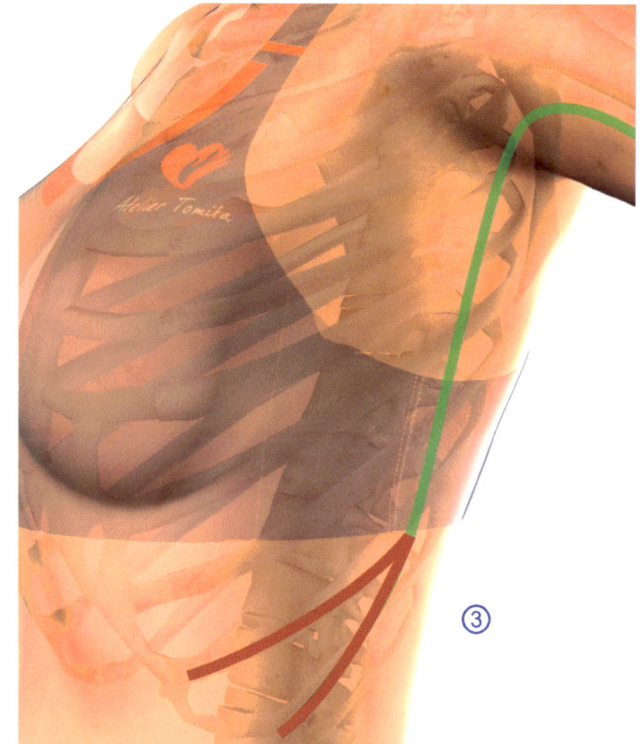

Treatment: STROKES

1. STROKE beneath the spine of the Scapula to medial, inferior
2. STROKE the Axillary border of the Scapula to inferior, lateral
3. STROKE the edge of the rib cage to anterior

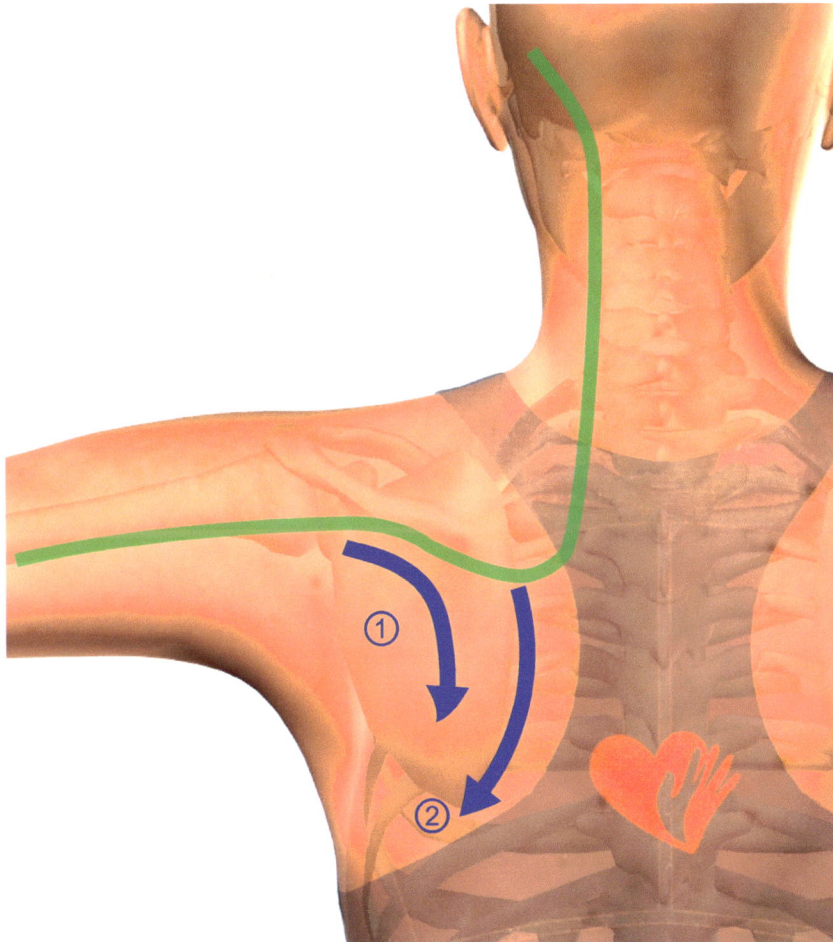

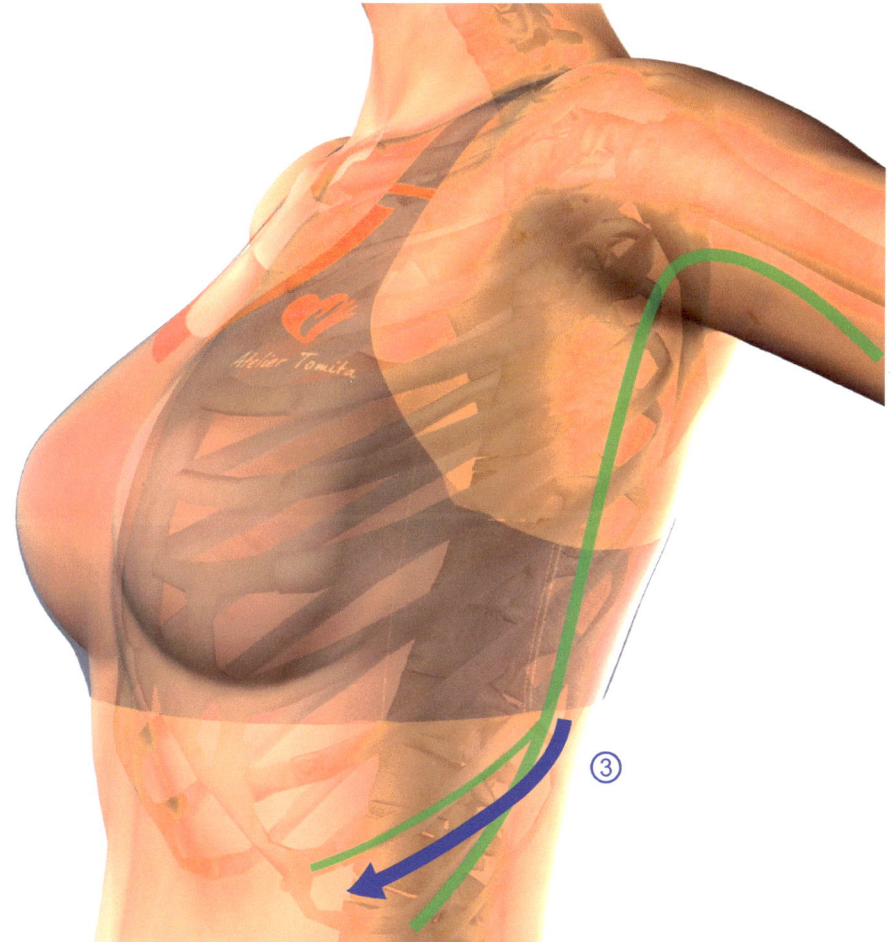

UNDERSTANDING OUR UNCONSCIOUS POSTURE

Most of the time the arm and frozen shoulder pain is caused by a very common bad sitting posture. People who work at a desk tend to bend forward with a rounded back, extended neck and cramped shoulders. Shoulder-blades are pulled up very high for extended periods of time. The weight of the arms is thus supported in suspension by the neck and the shoulder-blades.

People tend to unconsciously sit for long hours this way and it can lead to very painful tensions.

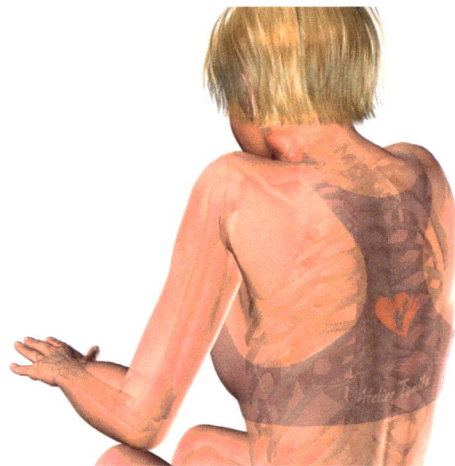

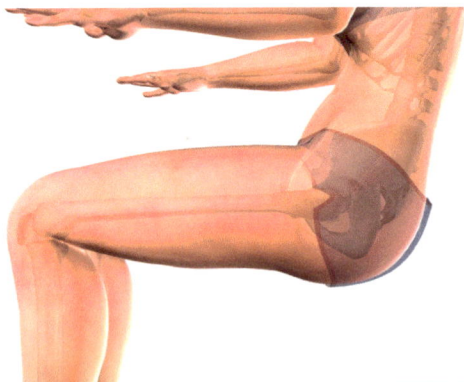

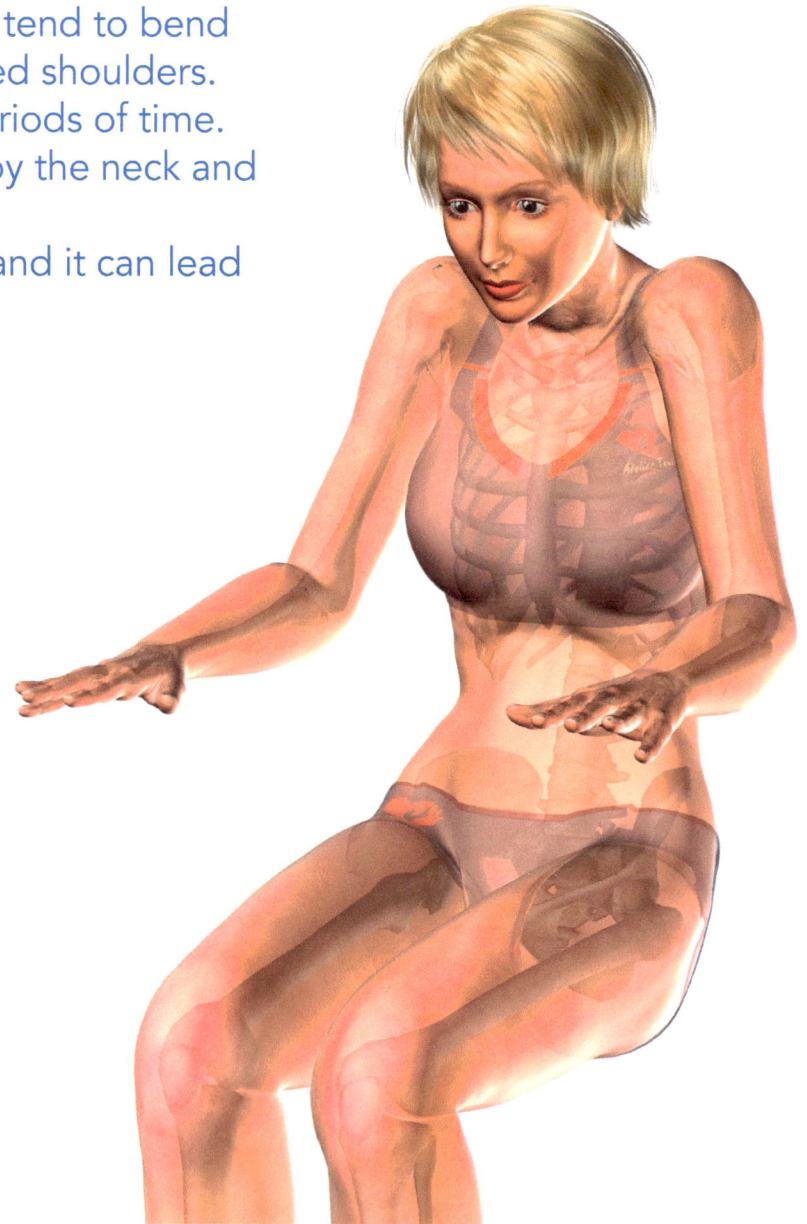

EFFECTIVE WAYS TO USE OUR ARMS

It is imperative to explain to the patient how to adopt a proper sitting posture. The most important is to release the weight of the shoulder-blades by rolling them up then backward so they sit flat in the back. The back-bone should be in an extended vertical line, up through the neck. It also helps to slide the buttocks toward the back of the chair. You should also advise the patient to adjust the height of their chair or desk in order to support the elbows.

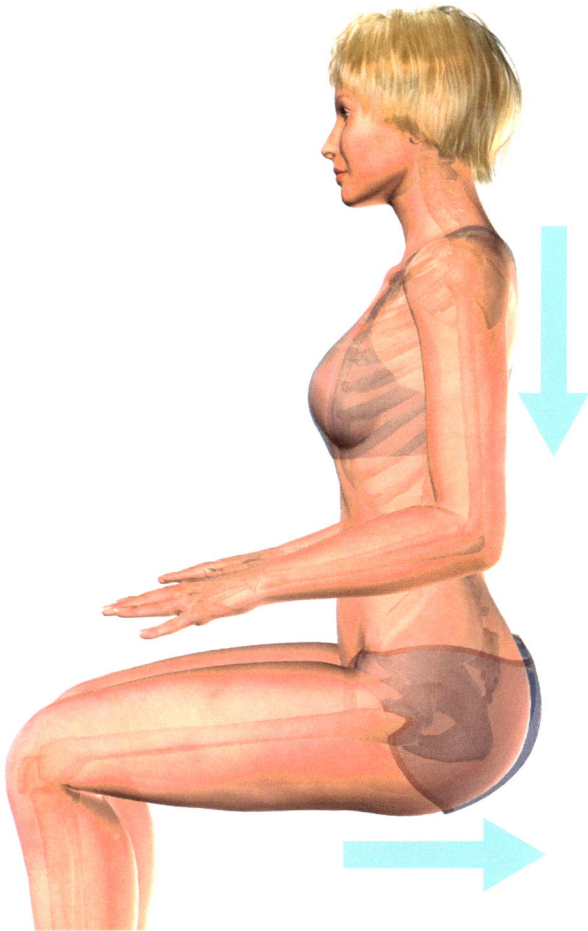

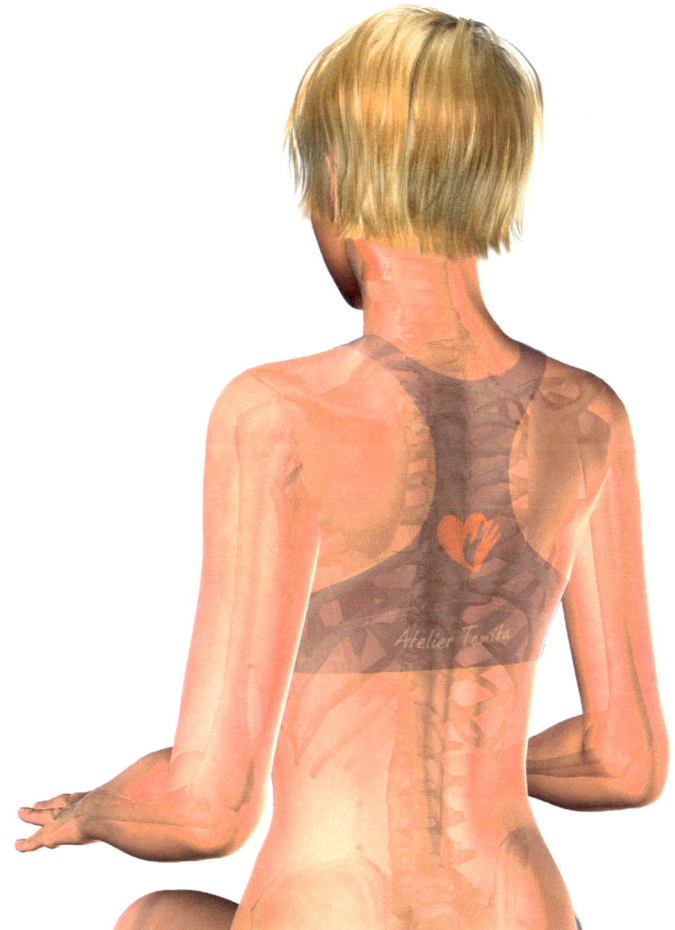

EVALUATION

1. Can you identify the 2 main myofascial tension lines related to arm and frozen shoulder pain?

2. Can you release the tension on the fingers?

3. Can you release the tension on the elbow?

4. Can you release the tension under the armpit?

5. Can you explain to your patient how to sit properly?

NOTES

LOWER BACK

OUTLINE

1. Understanding lower back pain
2. Releasing pain on center lower back and sacrum
   - Releasing tension on the big toe
   - Releasing tension inside the shin
   - Releasing tension inside the thigh
3. Releasing pain on lateral lower back and hip
   - Releasing tension on the fourth toe
   - Releasing tension outside the shin

UNDERSTANDING LOWER BACK PAIN

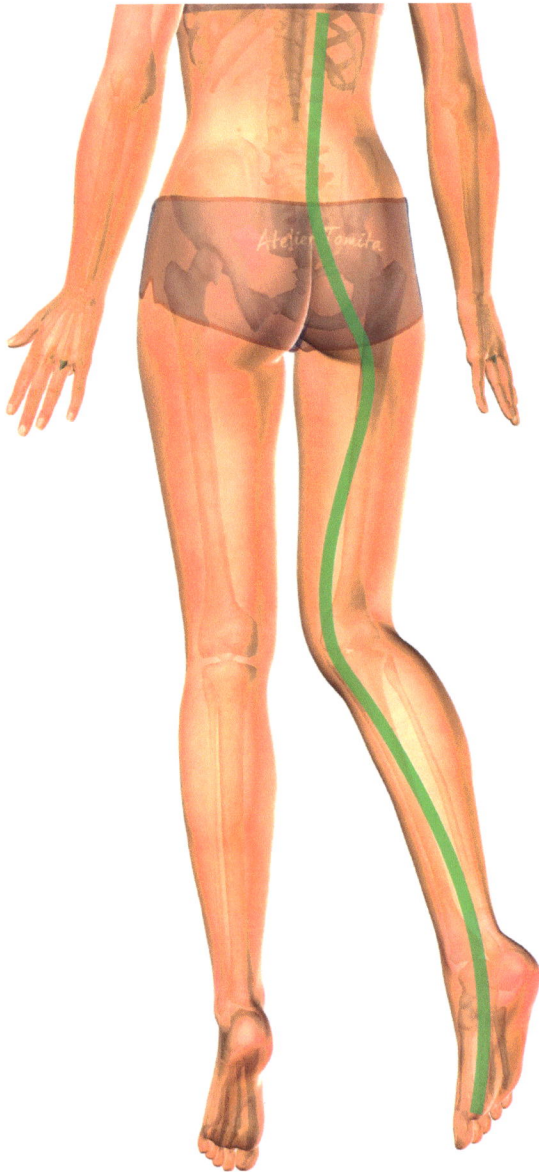

Mechanism:

The lower back is pulled by the myofascial connection to the legs. There are several specific connection lines on the legs, but we will focus here on the 2 basic ones: from the middle of the back and from the side of the hip. Identify the location of your patient's pain and apply proper treatments along the appropriate line. Even though they are basic, these will efficiently release tension in the lower back of your patient.

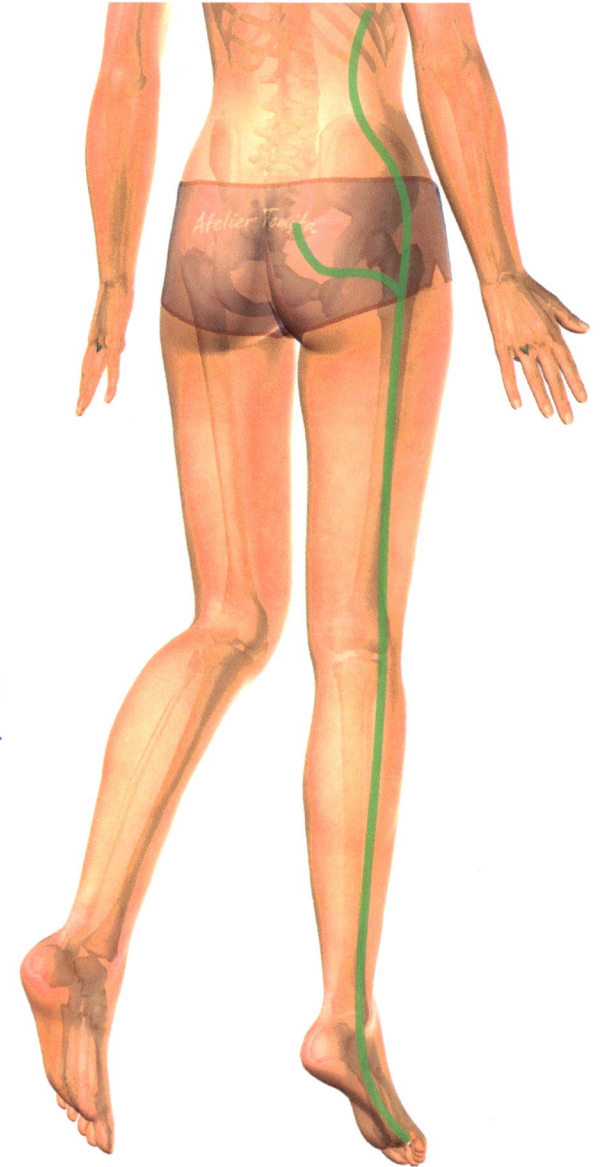

PAIN ON CENTER LOWER BACK AND SACRUM

PAIN ON LATERAL LOWER BACK AND HIP

RELEASING PAIN ON CENTER LOWER BACK AND SACRUM

Mechanism:

Posterior Foot Hallux Medial Line

When pain is concentrated in the middle of the lower back as shown on the picture, you should apply treatment along the myofascial tension line shown as the Green Line. The treatment points are on the bone edges marked in red.

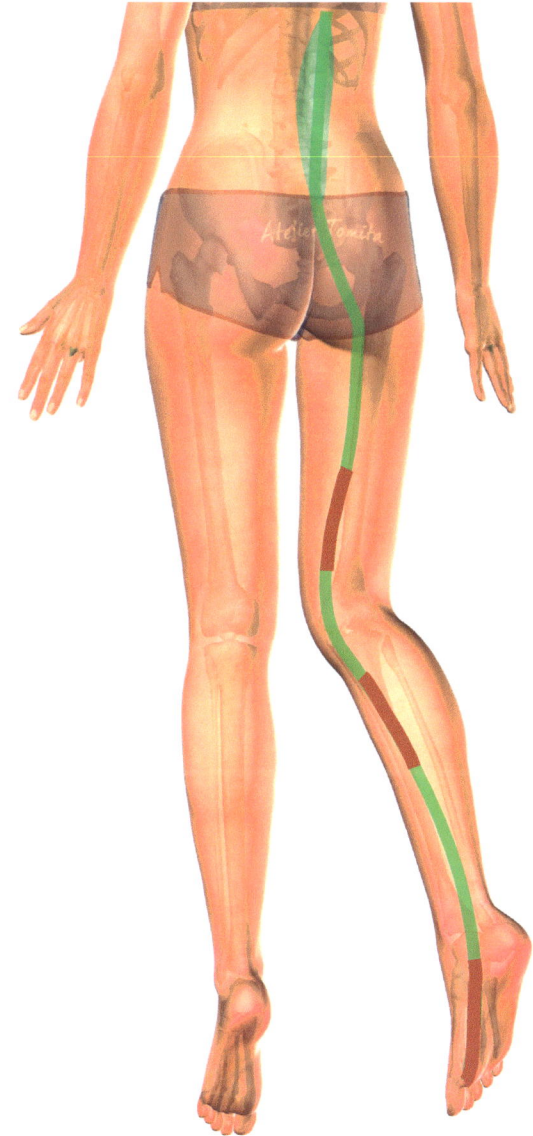

See also:
Superficial Back Line - Anatomy Train
Taiyang of foot meridian muscle - Jing jin

RELEASING TENSION ON THE BIG TOE

Treatment : SCRATCHES

1. SCRATCH the proximal edge of the proximal Phalange, medial side.
2. SCRATCH along the Metatarsal and SLIDE it to posterior
3. SCRATCH on the Calcaneus
4. SCRATCH around the Sesamoid bone
5. SCRATCH between Metatarsals

Some people are very ticklish on the feet. Carefully warn your patient that you will touch that area.

Some points are extremely painful as well. Check first if your strength is convenient to your patient. Adjust accordingly.

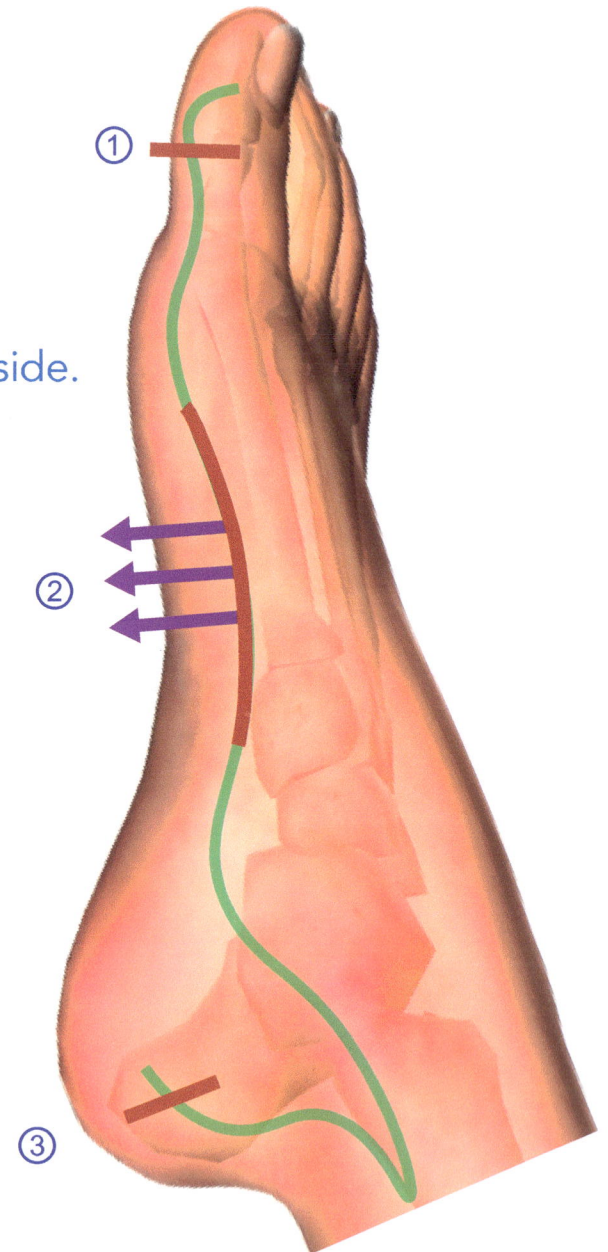

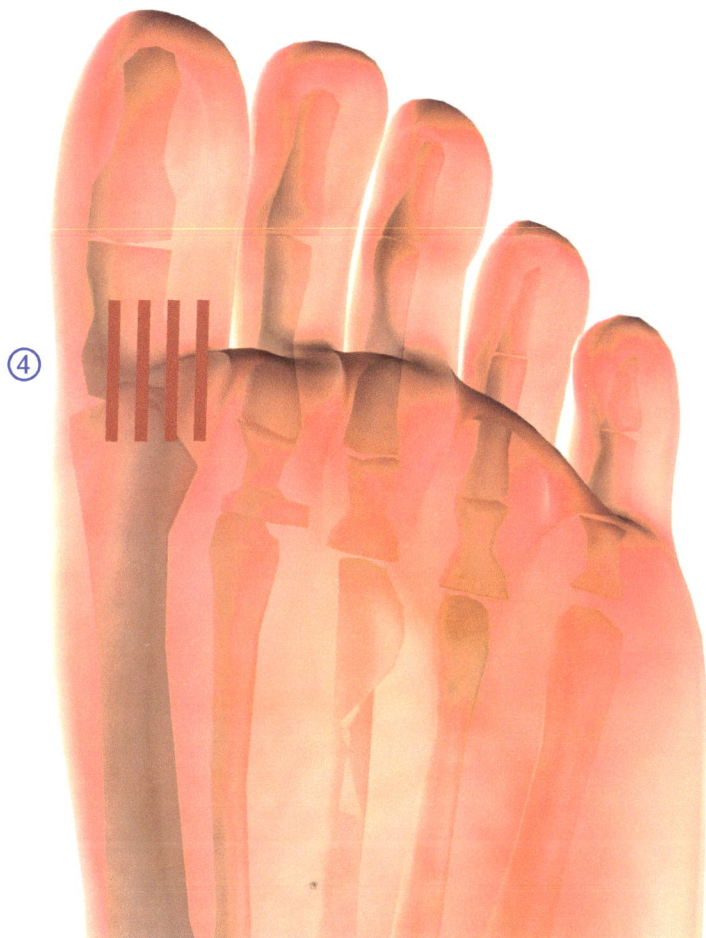

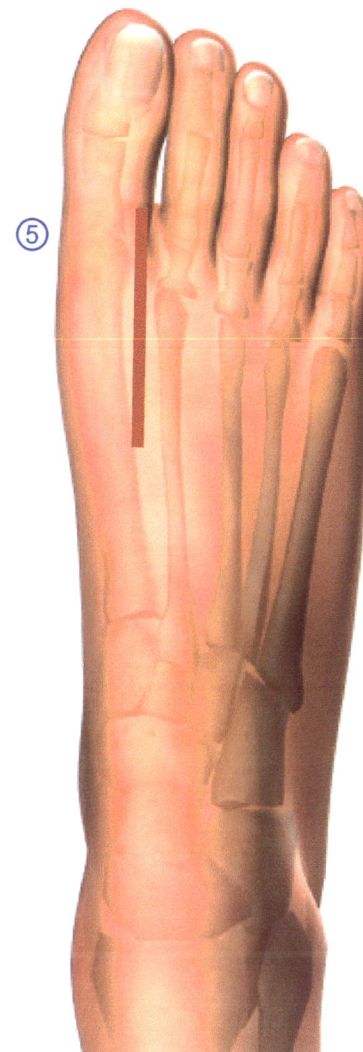

④

⑤

TIP!
Try to twist the Hallux gently to check the stiffness. Once the tension decrease, it will be easier to twist. Try to compare the stiffness on shin before/after this treatment. You may feel the difference!

RELEASING TENSION INSIDE THE SHIN

Treatment: SCRATCHES

1. SCRATCH the knee joint. (it's a narrow hollow)
2. SCRATCH along the proximal medial edge of the Tibia and SLIDE it to posterior

⚠️ Do not massage or apply strong pressure along the Red line at Point 2 ! This can cause internal-bleeding, inflammation or bruises.

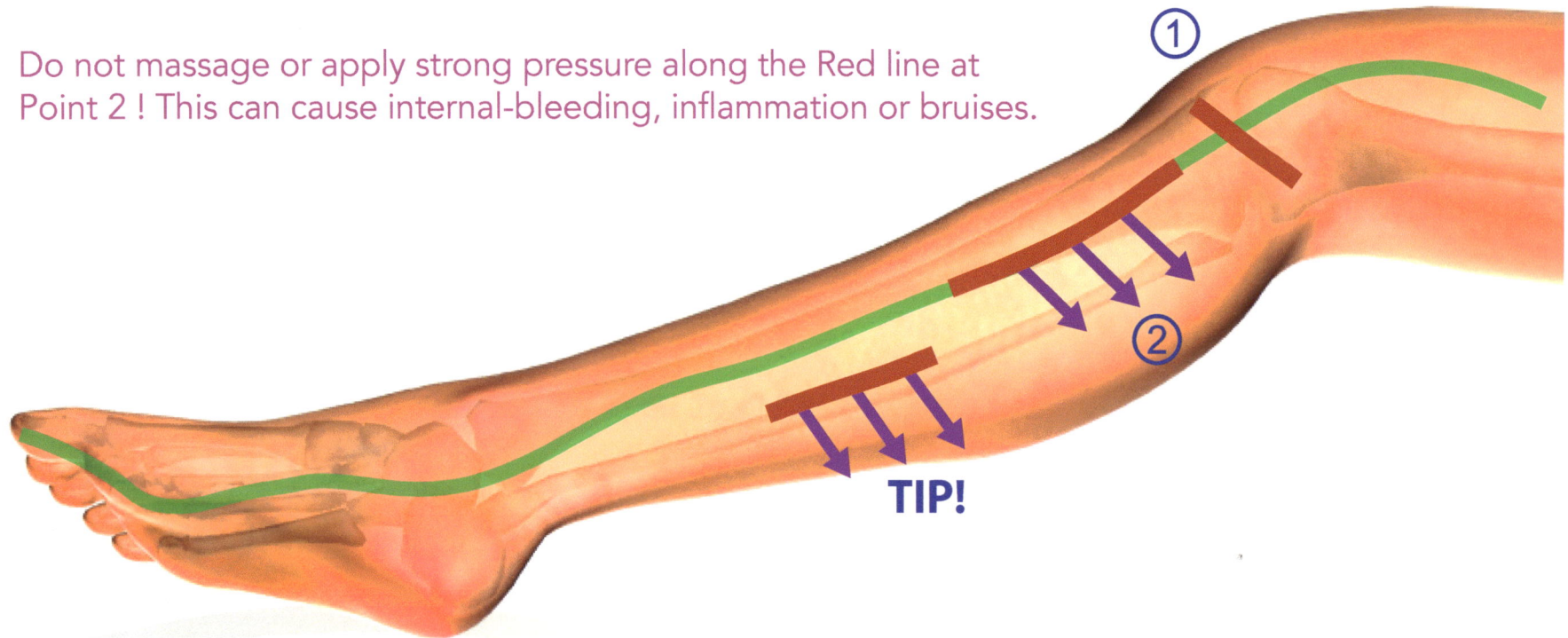

① ②

TIP!

TIP!
Find a tight thin string in the middle of the calf, SCRATCH along this string and SLIDE it to posterior. It can help prevent strained back!

Treatment: STROKES

1. STROKE along the Tibia upward.

This method can be used in combination with the scratches or alone when the patient is in too much pain. It is also an easy self-care technique to remember, especially for people with recurrent lower back pain.

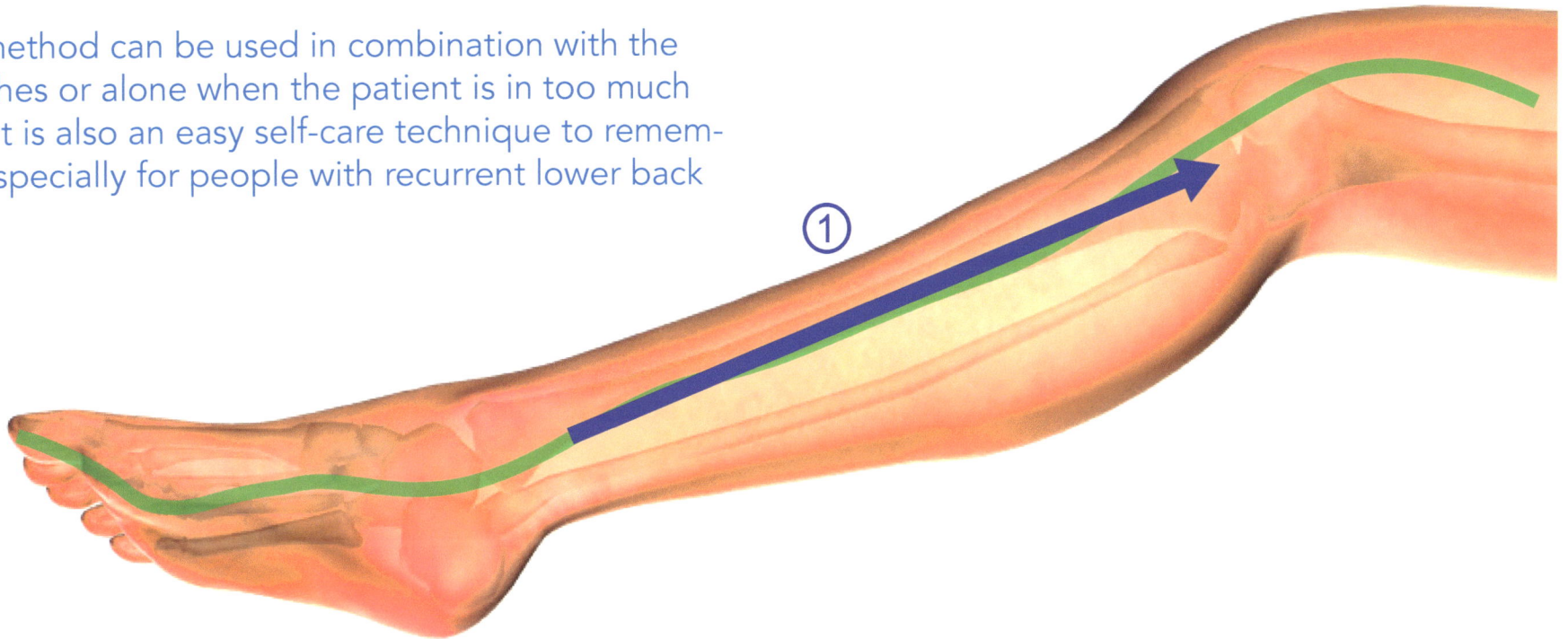

RELEASING TENSION INSIDE THE THIGH

Treatment: SCRATCHES

1. SCRATCH two lines as shown on the image
2. SCRATCH along the distal medial edge of the Femur and SLIDE it to posterior

⚠️ This area is very painful for most patients ! It is one of the typical hidden points of pain that the patients are unaware of.

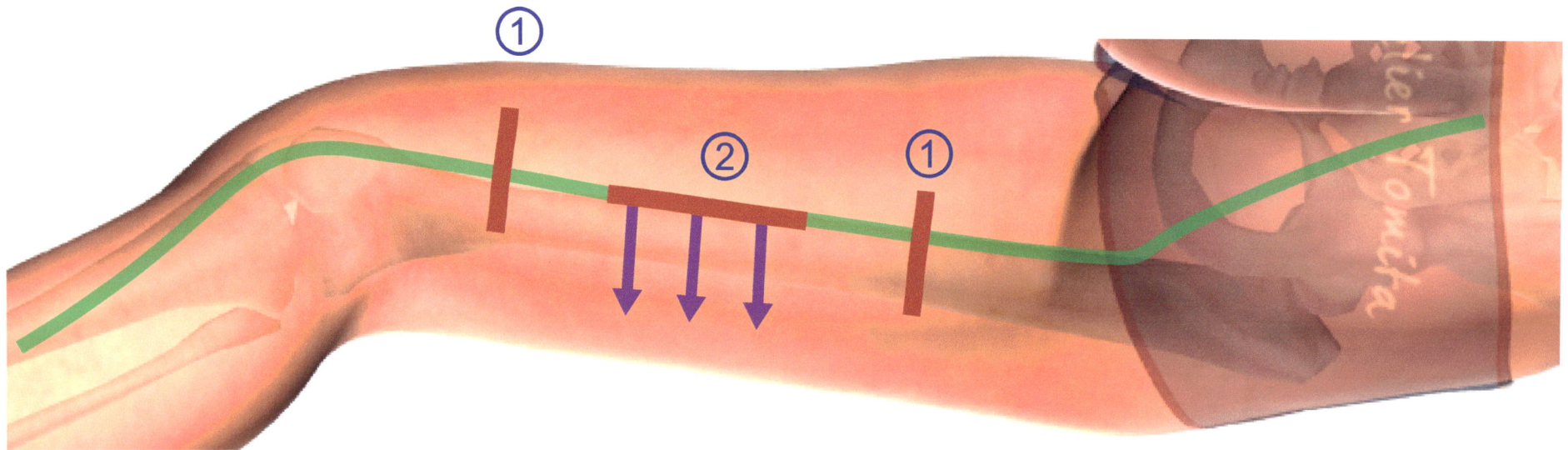

TIP!
This part is difficult to treat with your fingers because of the volume of the muscle. You can use your both thumbs or elbow. For self-care, your patient can sit in Yoga Easy Pose, and use their elbow to SLIDE this part.

Treatment: STROKES

1. STROKE medial thigh to posterior

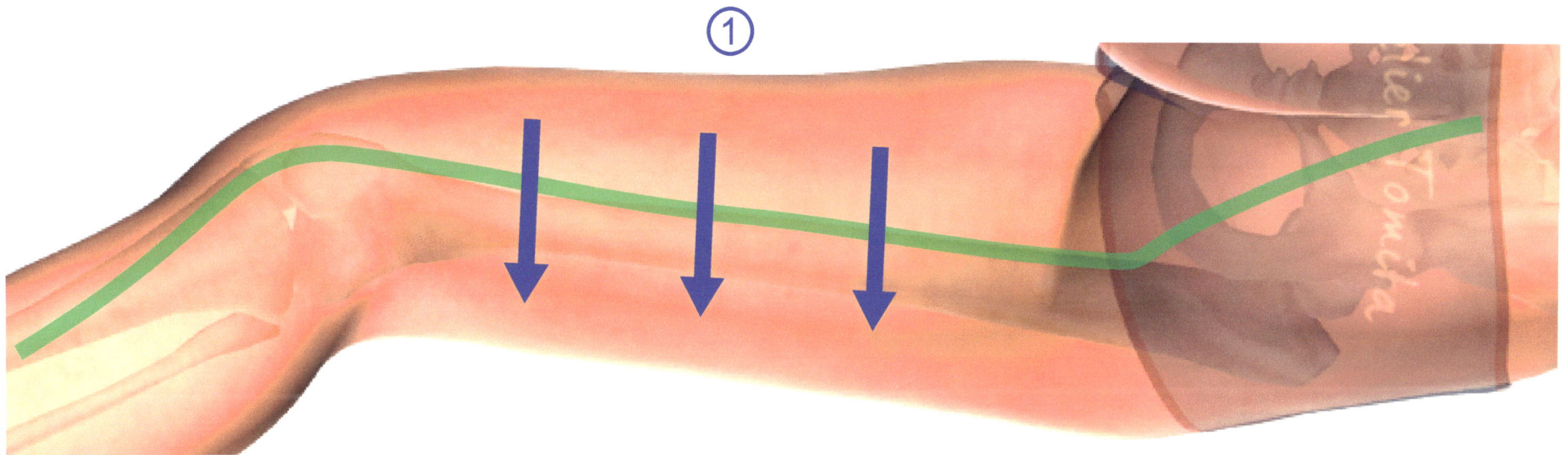

This method can be used as complement to the SCRATCHES, as it is a very difficult part to treat.

RELEASING PAIN ON LATERAL LOWER BACK AND HIP

Mechanism:

Posterior Foot 4th Lateral Line

When your patient feels pain on the side of the lower back or the side of the buttocks, apply your treatments along the myofascial tension line shown with the Green Line. The treatment points are on the bone edges marked in red.

See also:
Lateral Line - Anatomy Train
ShaoYang of foot meridian muscle - Jing jin

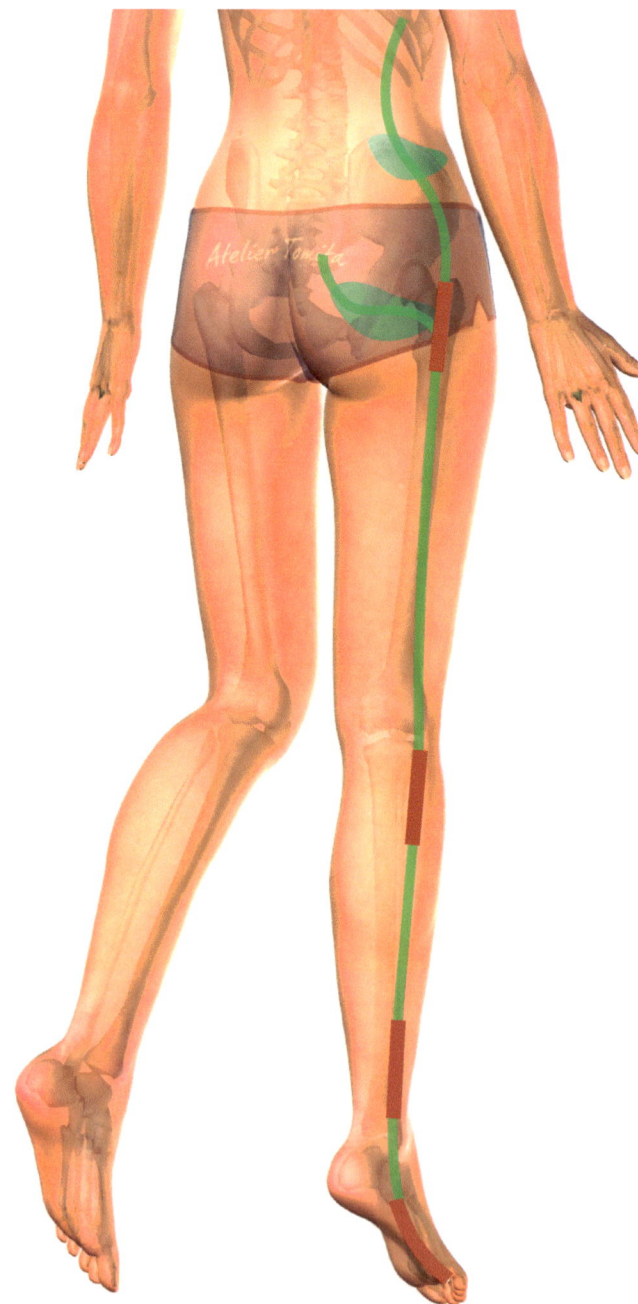

RELEASING TENSION ON THE FOURTH TOE

Treatment: SCRATCHES

1. SCRATCH the proximal edge of the proximal Phalange, lateral side.
2. SCRATCH the distal edge of the Metatarsal
3. SCRATCH between Metatarsals
4. PULL out the 5th proximal Phalange and then the 4th

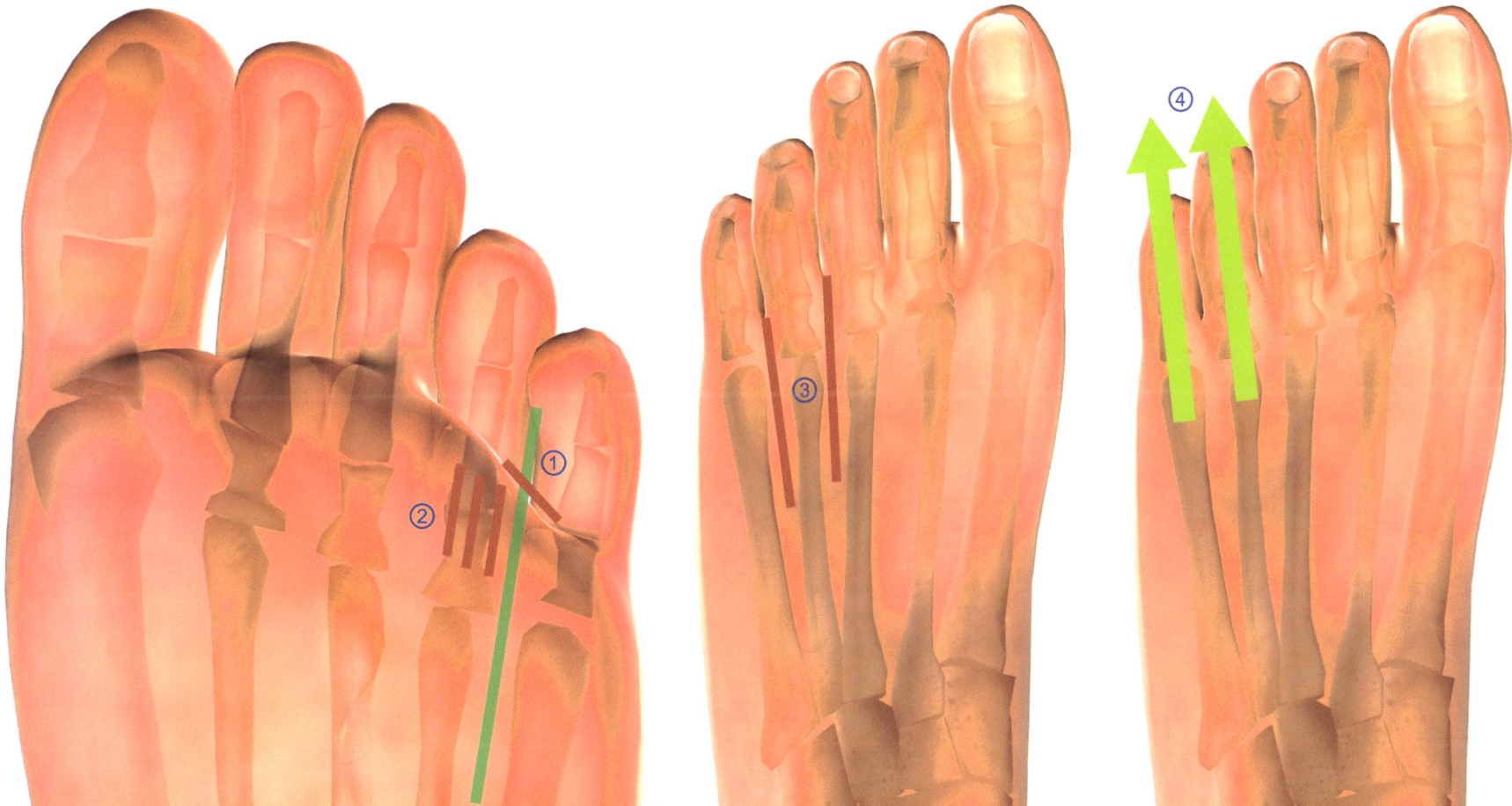

RELEASING TENSION OUTSIDE THE SHIN

Treatment: SCRATCHES

1. SCRATCH the proximal edge of the Fibula, lateral posterior side and SLIDE it to posterior

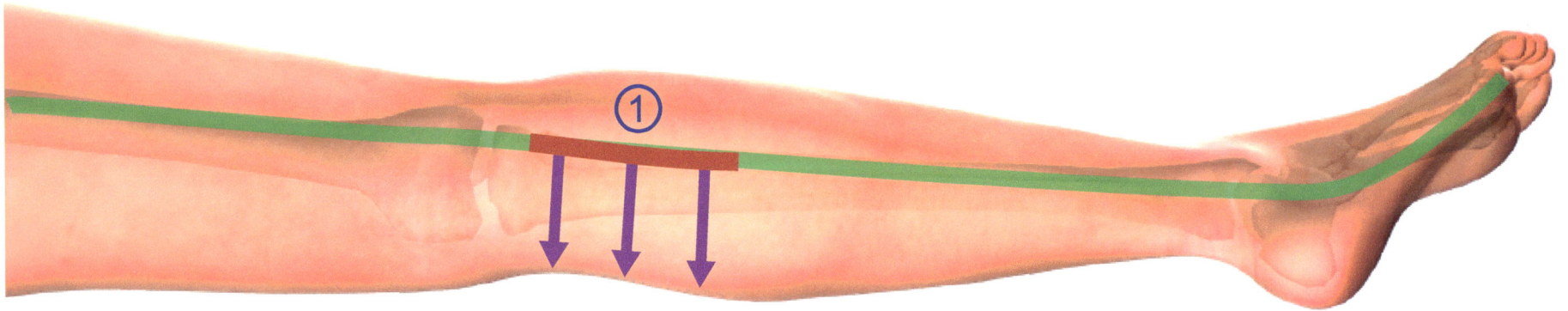

①

Treatment: STROKES

1. STROKE along the proximal edge of the Fibula upward

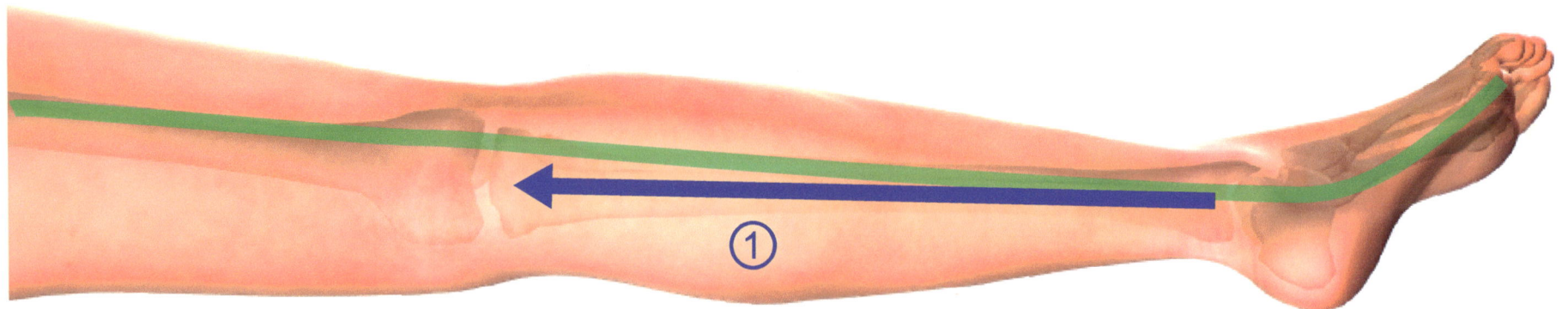

①

The **STROKES** method is recommended on patients that are experiencing extreme pain on their shin. It is also an easy self-care method for them to apply regularly.

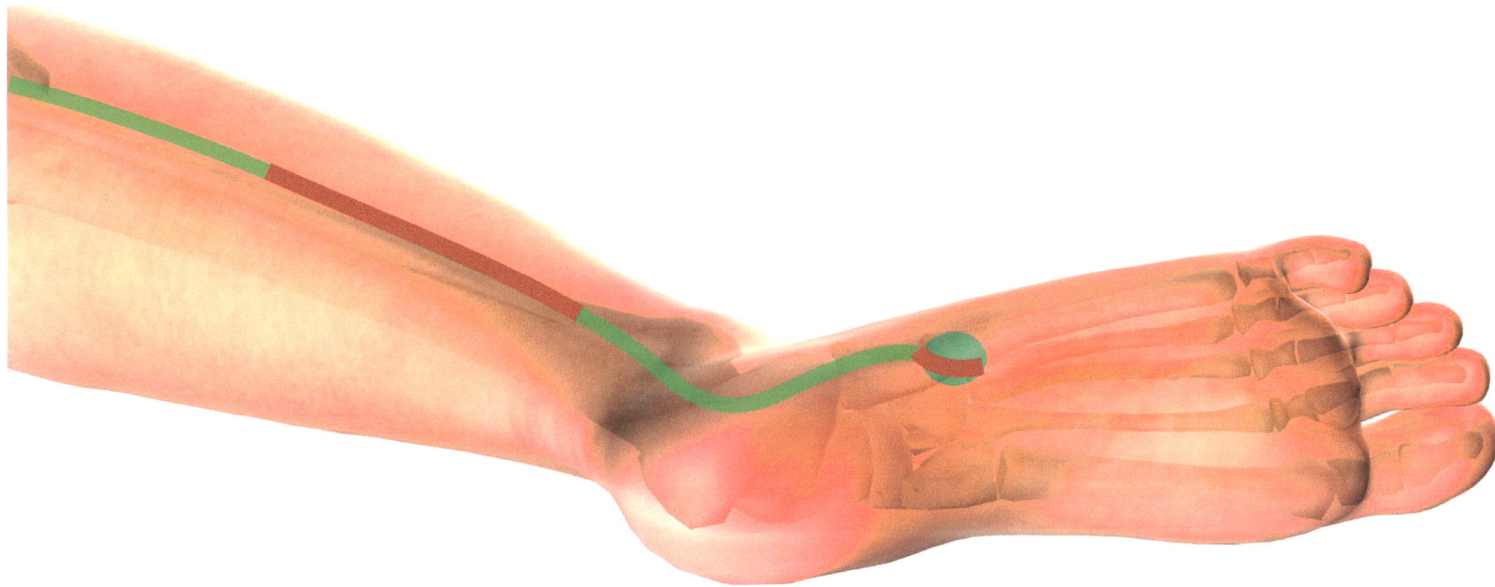

TIP!
When the distal edge of the Fibula is stiff, SCRATCH the posterior edge of the tuberosity of the 5th Metatarsal. (As shown in the picture above)

EVALUATION

1. Can you identify the two main myofascial tension lines to treat for lower back pain?

2. Can you release tension on toes?

3. Can you release tension on th shin?

4. Can you release tension on the thigh?

5. What self-care methods would you recommend to your patient?

NOTES

KNEE

OUTLINE

1. Understanding knee pain
2. Releasing pain deep inside the knee
   - Releasing tension on the Achilles tendon
   - Releasing tension on the calf
   - Releasing tension on the Sacrum
3. Releasing pain beneath the knee
   - Releasing tension on the dorsum of the foot
   - Releasing tension on the thigh
   - Releasing tension on the Ilium
   - Releasing tension on the chest

UNDERSTANDING KNEE PAIN

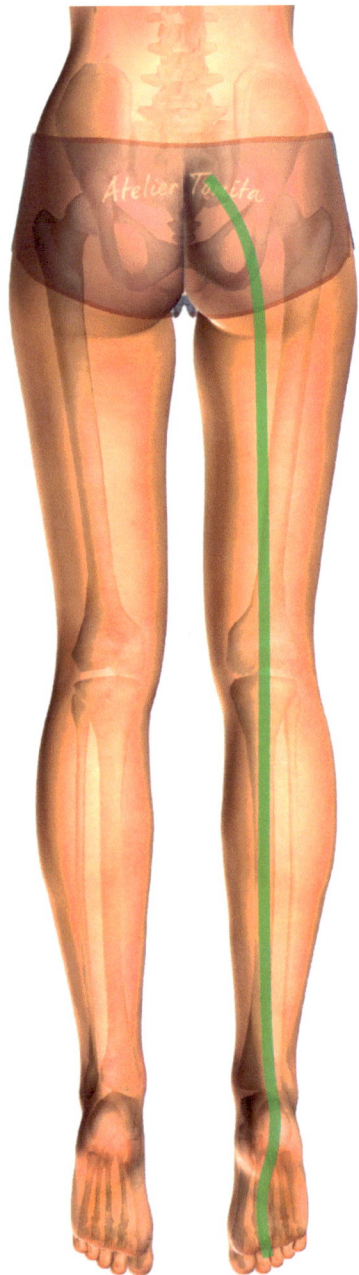

Mechanism:

Knee pain is a very complex problem and can come from various origins. The myofascial tension lines stretch from both the front of the body and the back of the body.

When the pain seems to come from deep inside the knee, we will apply treatment along the line that connects the sacrum to the toes.

When the pain seems to be located rather beneath the knee, we will apply treatment along the line that stretches from as far up as the chest, to down to the tip of the toes.

The knee is a very delicate that is easy to damage. Do NOT put any pressure on, behind or around the knee. This can cause further injuries to your patient. As always, start your treatments from the farthest ends of the myofascial tension lines.

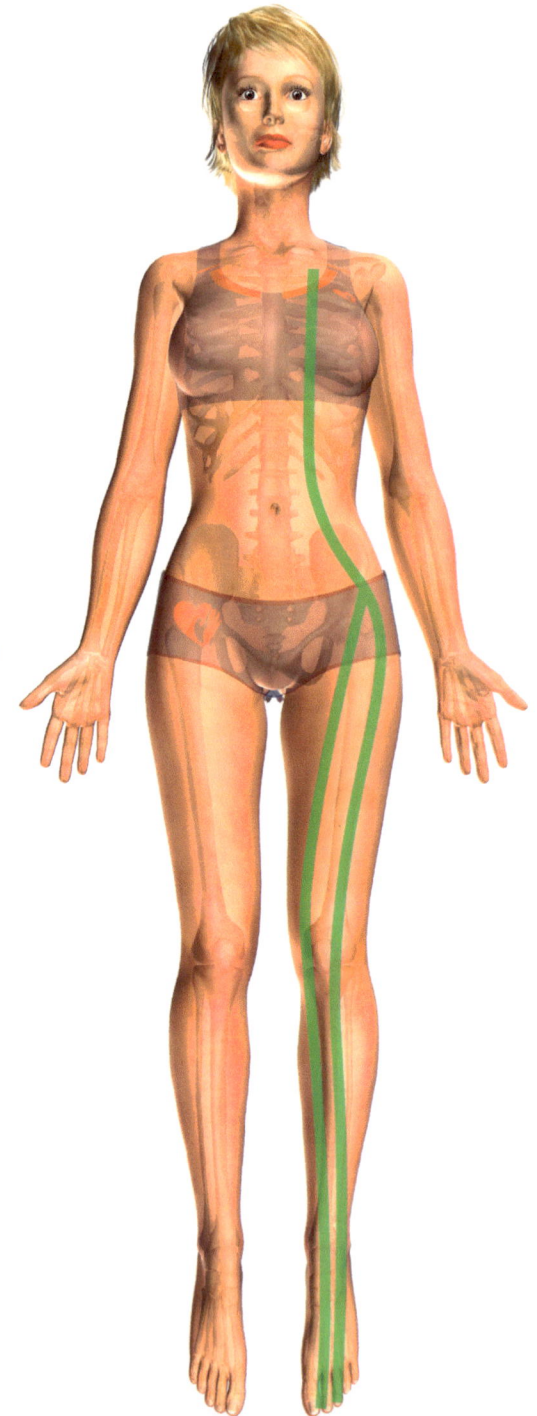

RELEASING PAIN DEEP INSIDE THE KNEE

Mechanism:

Posterior Foot Long Lateral Line

If your patient's knee pain seems to be located rather inside the knee, you should apply your treatments along the myofascial tension line that stretches between the sacrum and the long toe of that side of the body, as shown with the Green Line on the picture. The treatment points are located on the bone edges marked in red.

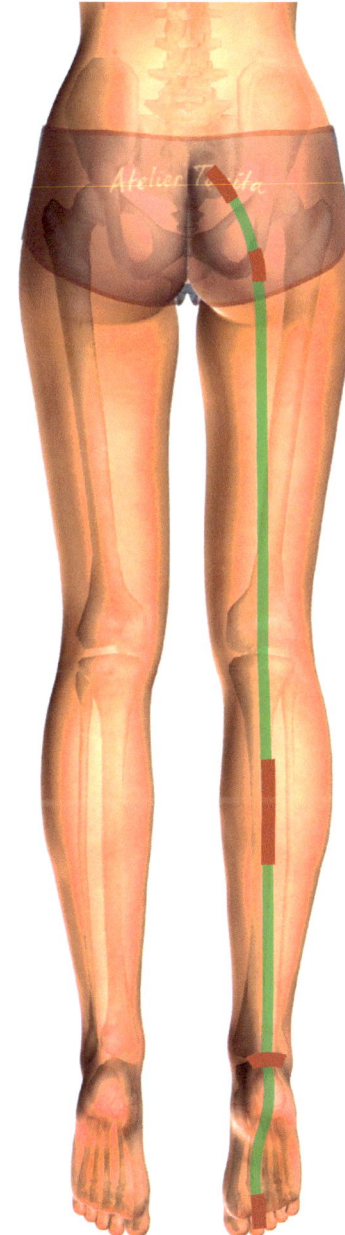

See also:
Superficial Back Line - Anatomy Train
Taiyang of foot meridian muscle - Jing jin

RELEASING TENSION ON THE ACHILLES TENDON

Treatment: SCRATCHES

1. SCRATCH the proximal edge of the proximal Phalange, lateral side.
2. SCRATCH the distal edge of the Metatarsal
3. SCRATCH between Metatarsals
4. SCRATCH the proximal edge of the Calcaneus and SLIDE the Achilles tendon to lateral direction

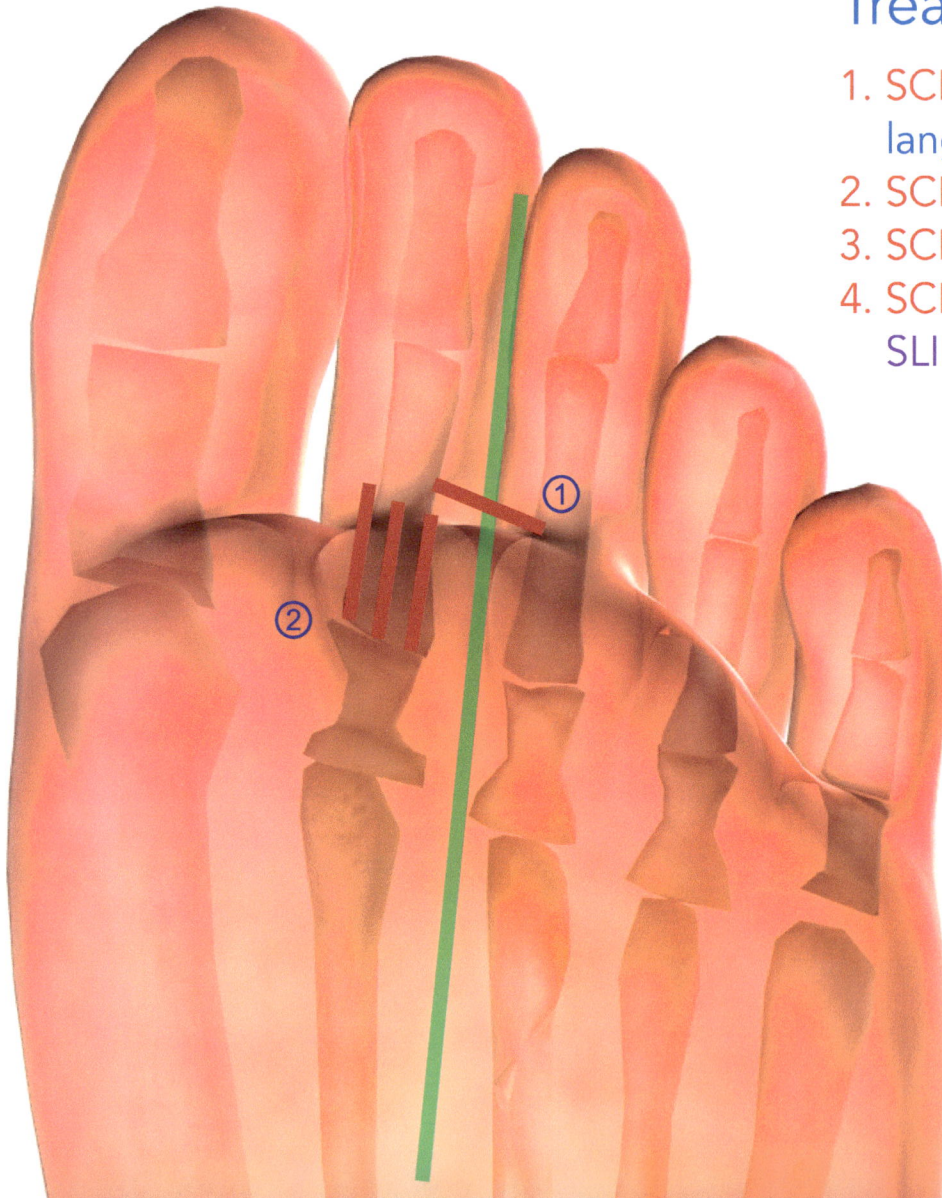

The Achilles tendon is a very delicate part of the foot. Do NOT pull it NOR scratch directly onto it. This could cause very severe injuries.

Some people have very stiff Achilles tendons. Do not over work on this area.

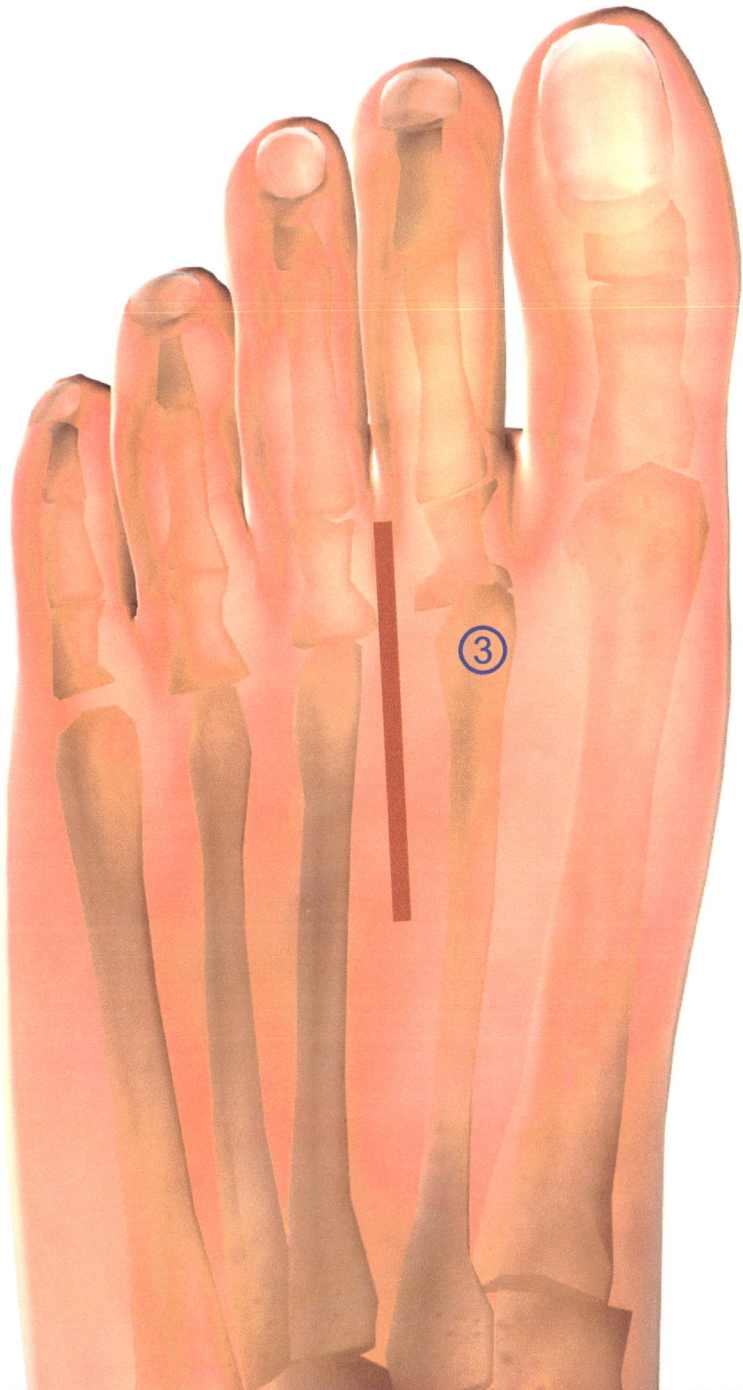

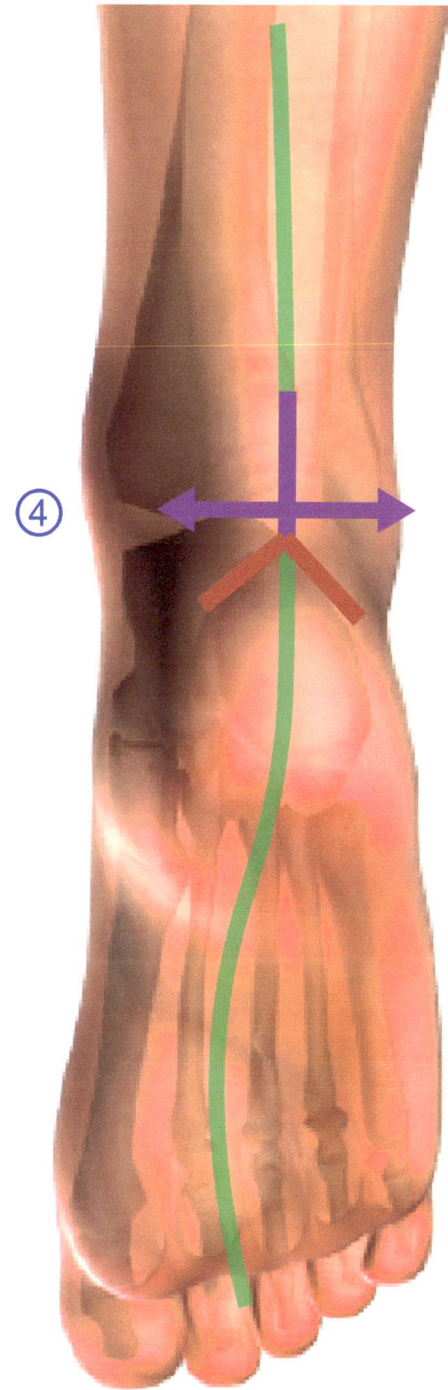

③

④

RELEASING TENSION ON THE CALF

Treatment: SCRATCHES

1. SCRATCH the center of the calf, the proximal edge, and SLIDE it to lateral.
2. SCRATCH the middle of the calf from distal to proximal, and SLIDE all to lateral.

⚠️ Some people have very stiff and numb calves, as others, especially athletes, might have very sensitive tight calves. Be very gentle in your approach and adjust your strength to the patient's sensitiveness. If pain is too acute, use only the STROKES method.

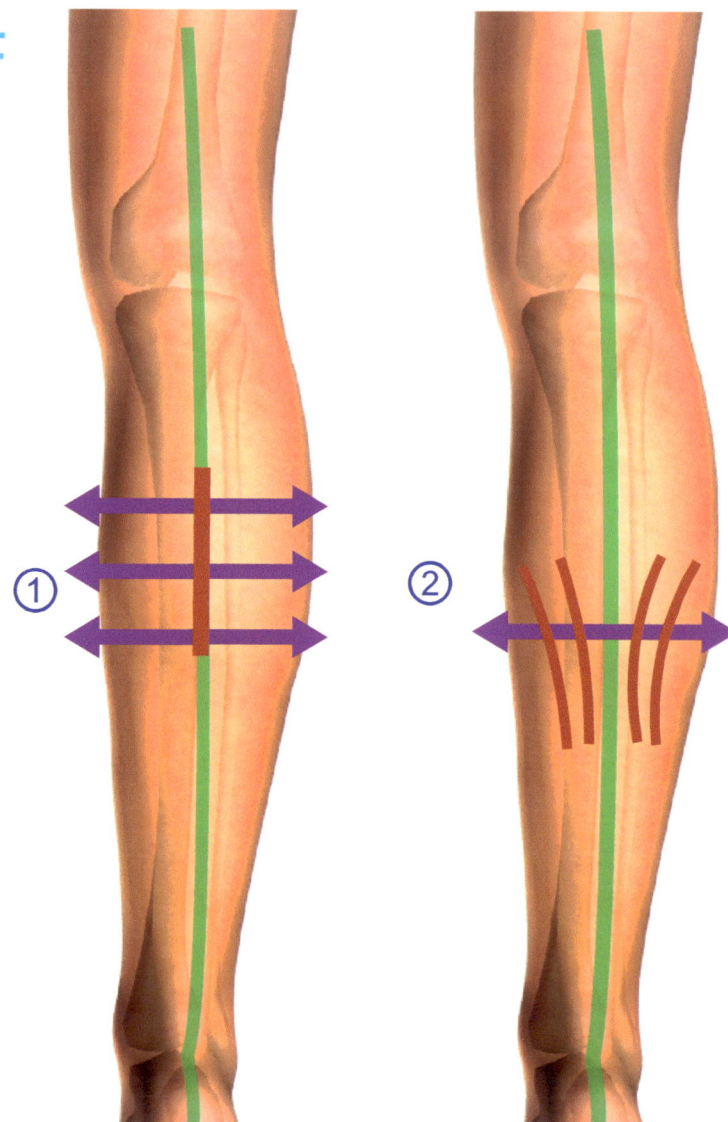

① ②

TIP!

1. Find the hollow between the 2 heads of the Gastrocnemius, and SCRATCH along it. You may find some stiffness in the deep, posterior lateral side of the Tibia

2. Climb up the swelling of the Gastrocnemius. SCRATCH several lines on all sides of calf.

Treatment: STROKES

1. STROKE the center of the calf downward, and STROKE medial/lateral

①

You can use the STROKES method as a first approach to very sensitive calves, and switch to the SCRATCHES when the tension starts to release. This technique is also a good one to teach to your patient as self-care maintenance.

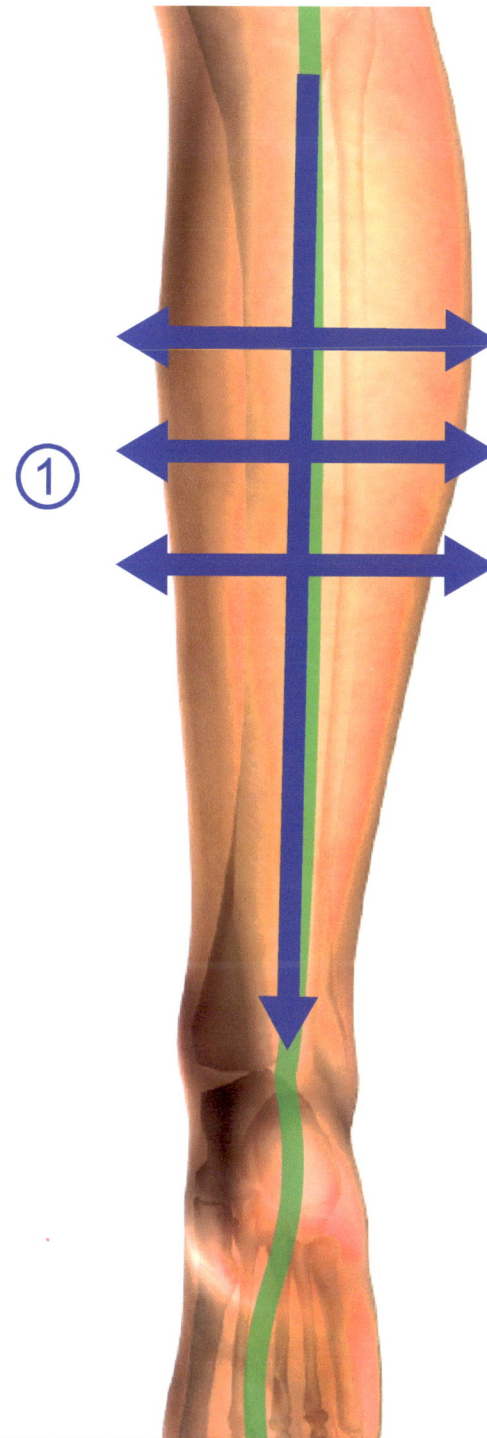

RELEASING TENSION ON THE SACRUM

Treatment: SCRATCHES

1. SCRATCH along the hollow lateral side of the Sacrum and SLIDE it to lateral
2. SCRATCH on the Ischium

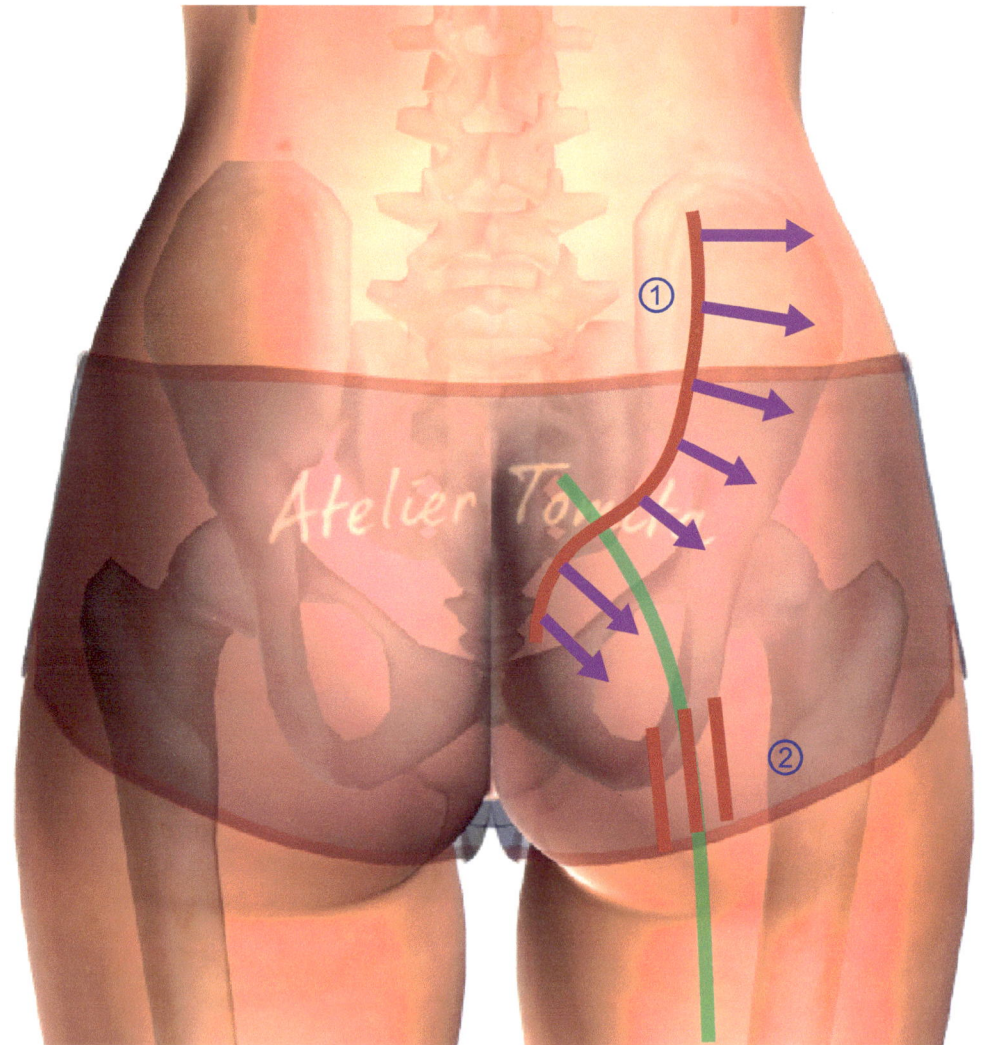

These points are close to the Anus and Genitals.

⚠️ A polite explanation is necessary before the treatment.

Double check that all the parts are covered with cloth before touching.

RELEASING PAIN BENEATH THE KNEE

Mechanism:

If you evaluate that the pain is located rather beneath the knee, you should apply treatment along the front myofascial tension lines that connect the chest all the way down to the toes:

The Anterior Foot Long Medial Line and
The Anterior Foot Long Lateral Line

The main myofascial tension lines divides at the hip in two main lines along the leg, a shown with the Green Lines. The treatment points are located on the bone edges marked in red.

See also:
Superficial Front Line - Anatomy Train
YangMing of foot meridian muscle - Jing jin

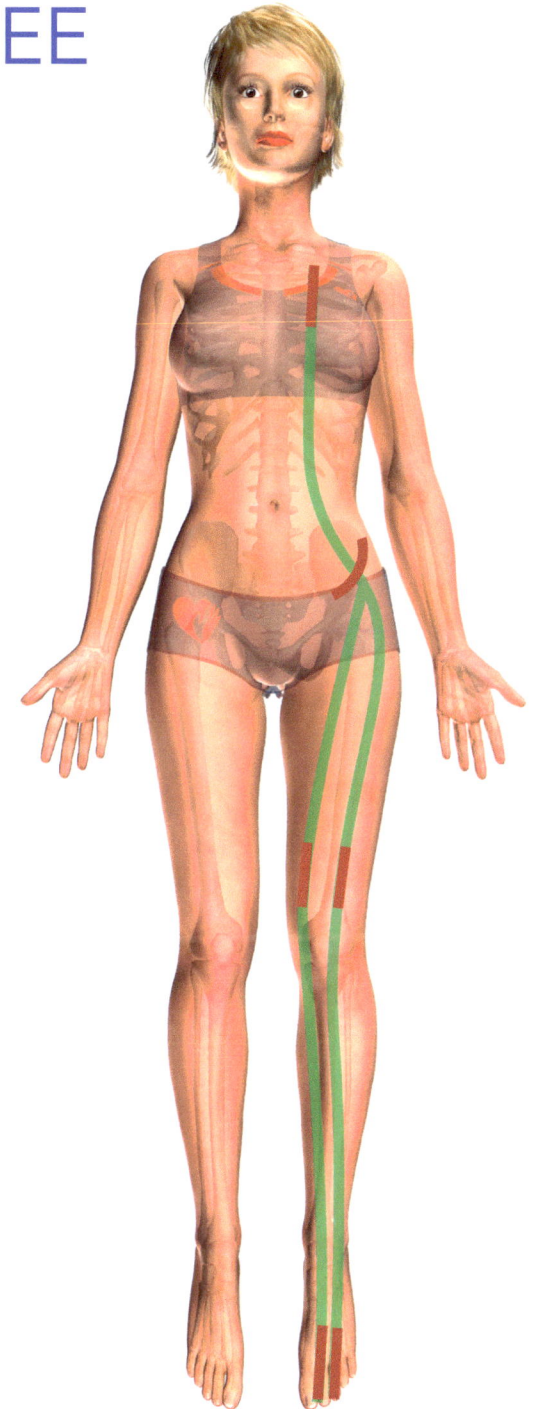

RELEASING TENSION ON THE DORSUM OF THE FOOT

Treatment: SCRATCHES

1. SCRATCH between Metatarsals

⚠️ People with very stiff feet will find this very uncomfortable, sometimes painful. Be very gentle or simply move the foot with your both hands.

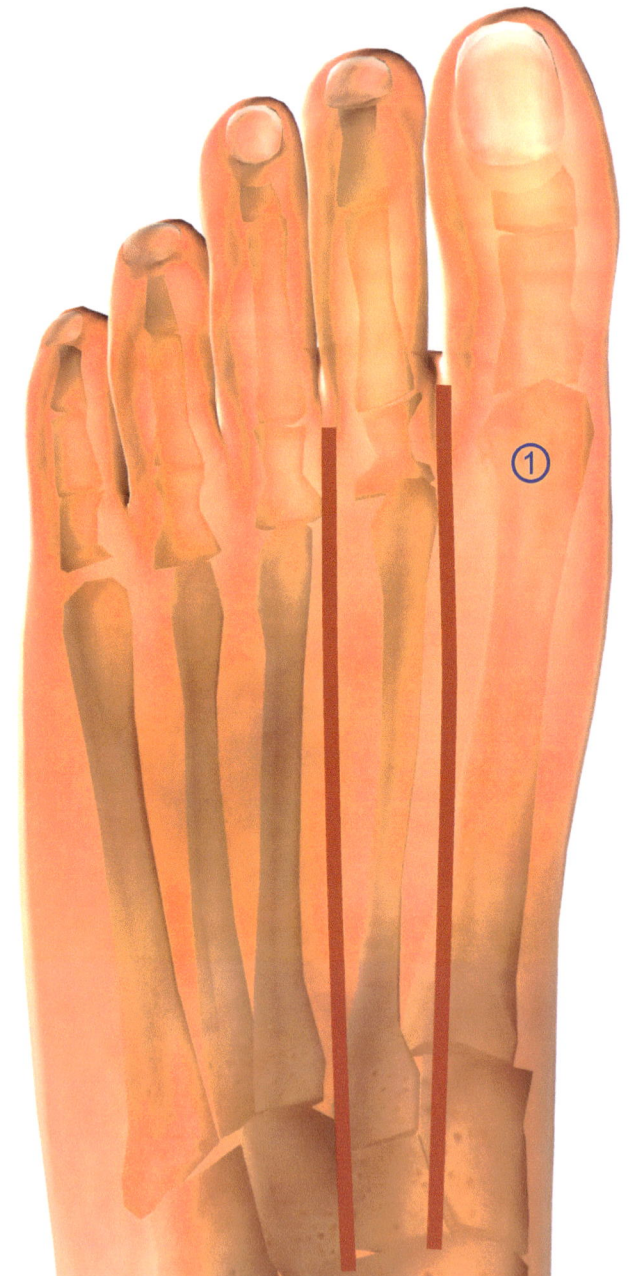

①

RELEASING TENSION ON THE THIGH

Treatment: SCRATCHES

1. SCRATCH the distal medial edge of the Femur and SLIDE it to Medial
2. SCRATCH the distal lateral edge of the Femur and SLIDE it to Lateral

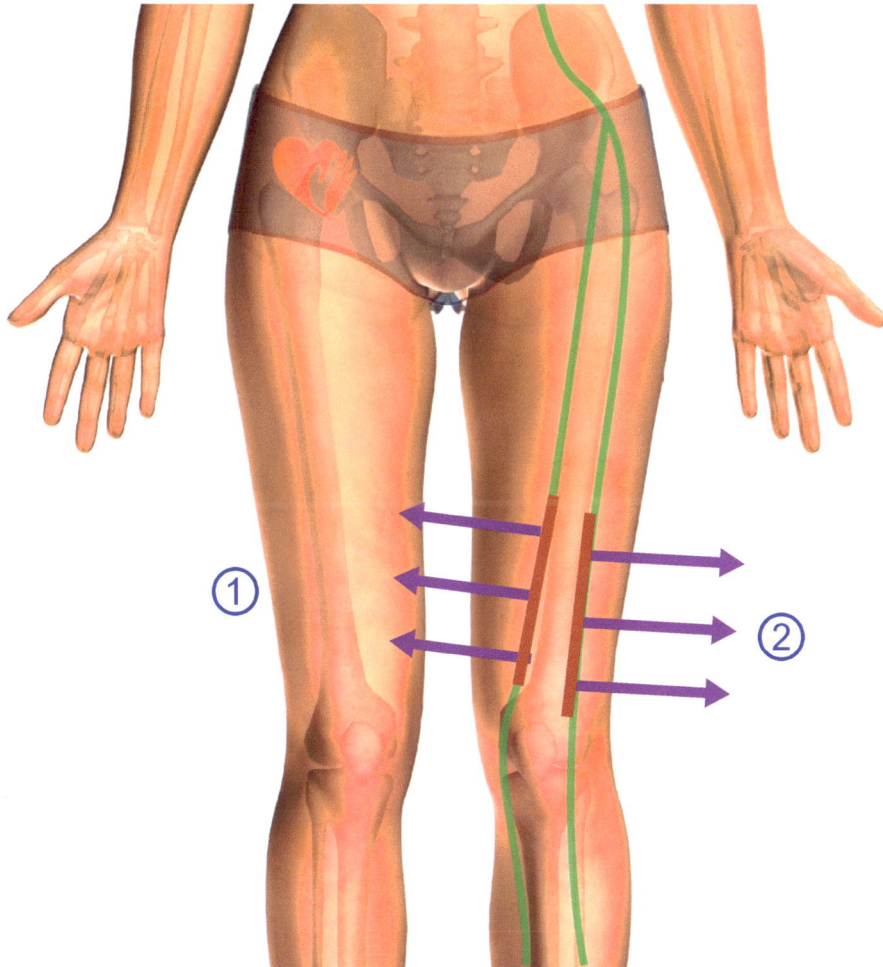

Treatment: STROKES

1. STROKE along the Femur upward and medial/lateral from the Femur

Ticklish people will prefer the STROKES technique. It is also useful for sef-care.

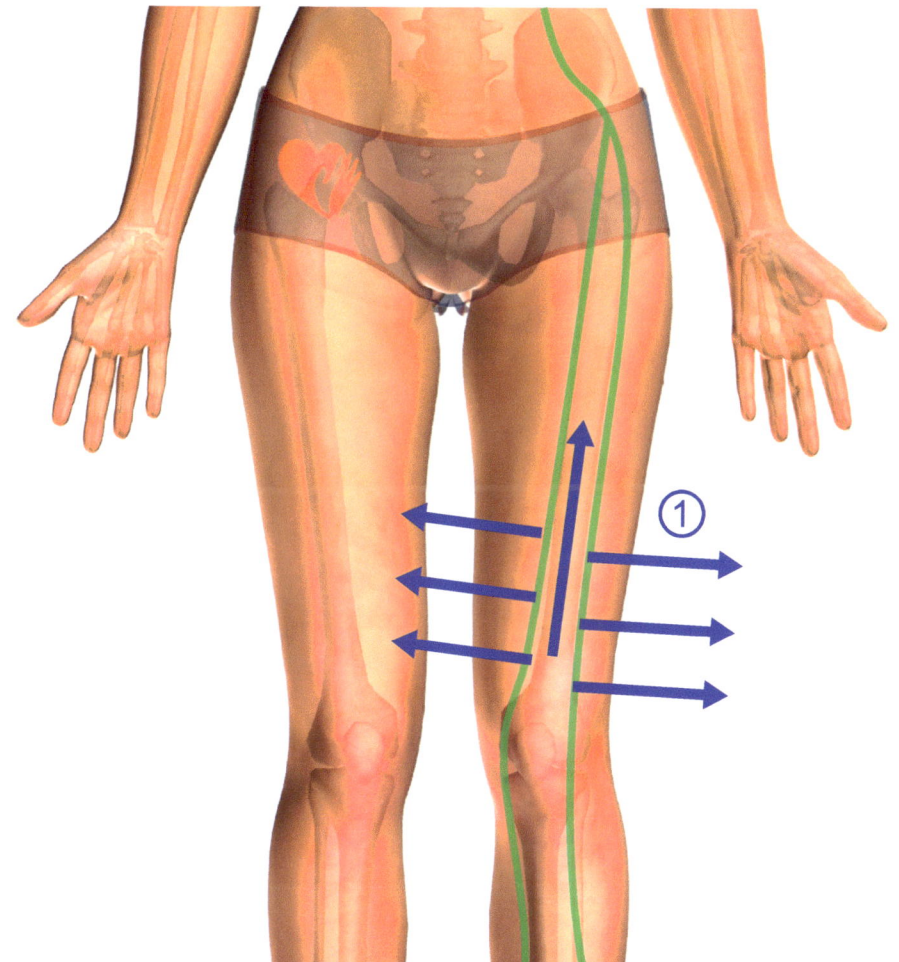

RELEASING TENSION ON THE ILIUM

Treatment:

1. Touch the edge of the Ilium and SLIDE it to inside

⚠️ Don't push in strongly to the abdominal organs.

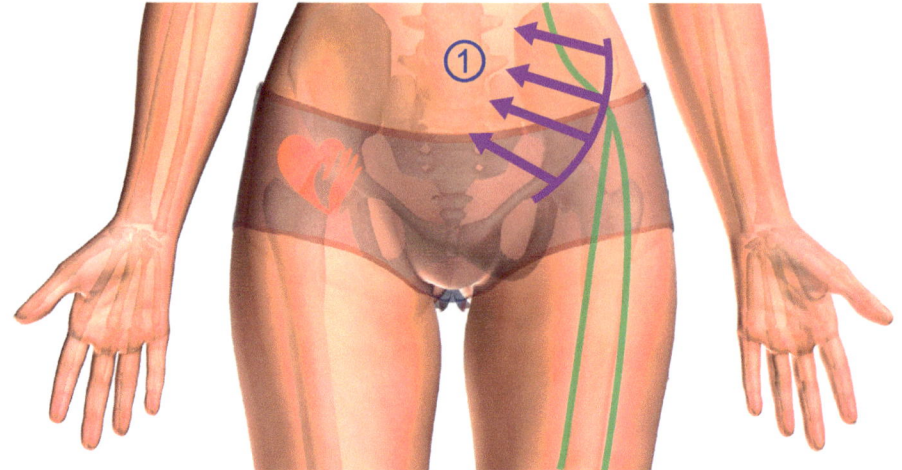

Treatment: STROKES

1. STROKE the inferior edge of the Ilium to medial
2. STROKE the superior edge of the Ilium to lateral

⚠️ This is a very delicate zone and some patients will be uncomfortable with being touched around the abdominal area. Give explanations before you start the treatment. You can teach reluctant patients how to perform this by themselves.

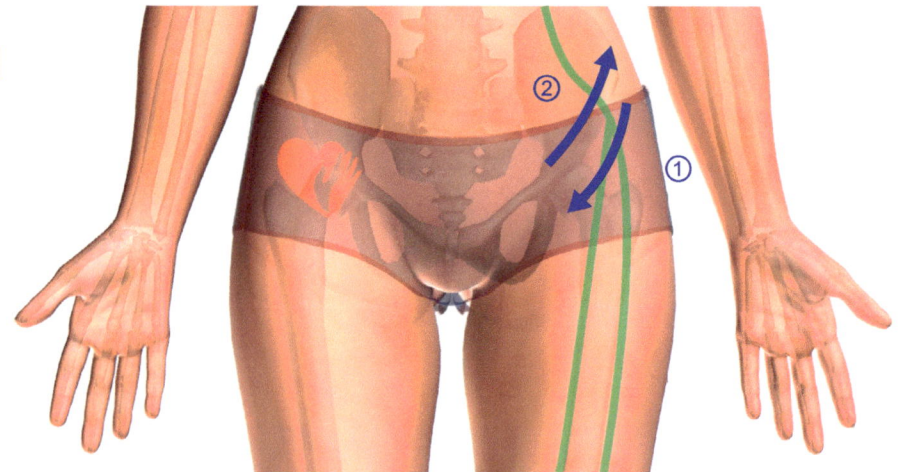

RELEASING TENSION ON THE CHEST

Treatment:

1. Imagine the green square, and SLIDE it to lateral

⚠️ This is usually slightly painful when performed for the first time. Explain to your patient that this will go away very quickly and that the pain will not come back for a long while.

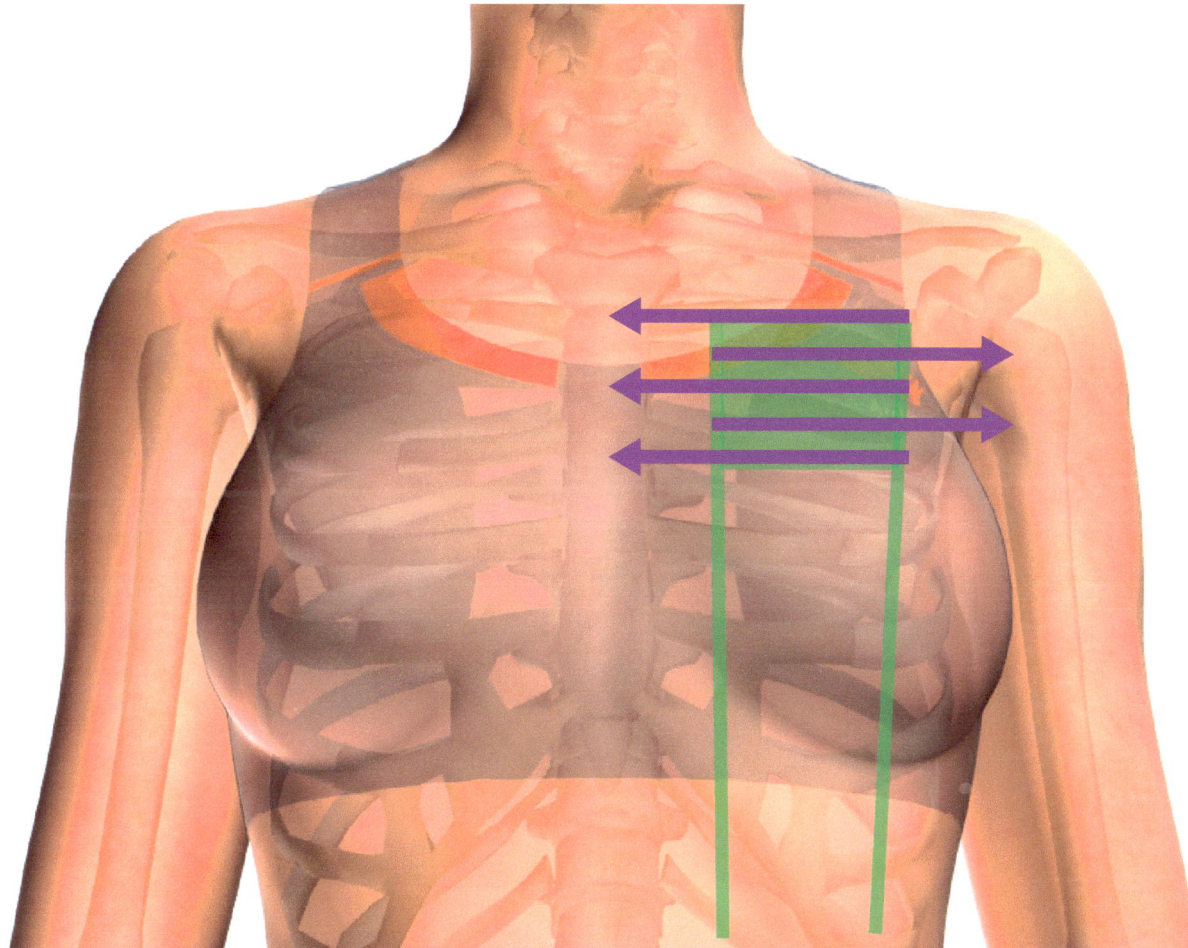

EVALUATION

1. Can you explain the two main mechanisms of the knee pain-related myofascia tension lines?

2. Can you release tension on the Achilles tendon and the calf?

3. Can you release tension on the sacrum?

4. Can you release tension on the thigh and Ilium?

5. What can you teach your patient for self-care?

NOTES

ABDOMEN AND BACK

OUTLINE

1. Understanding tension on the abdomen and the back
2. Releasing tension on the abdomen
   - Releasing tension on the Ilium edge
   - Releasing tension on the Pubis edge
   - Releasing tension on the Rectus Abdominis
3. Releasing back tension
   - Releasing tension on the Erector Spinae
   - Releasing tension on the intercostal muscle
   - Releasing tension on the Sacrum

UNDERSTANDING TENSION ON THE ABDOMEN AND THE BACK

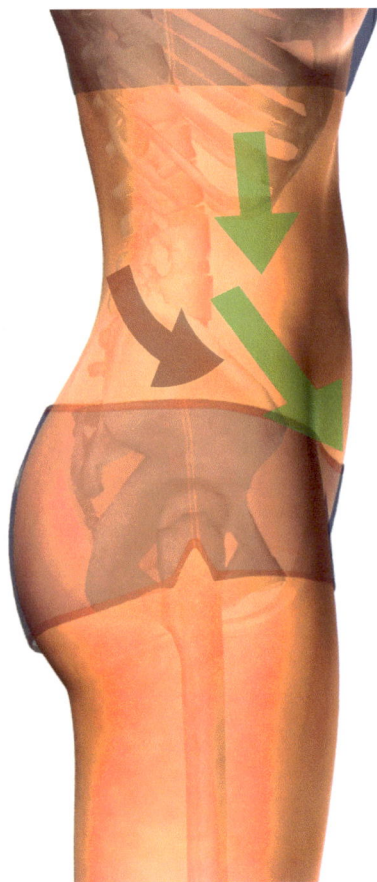

Mechanism:

Digestive stress causes the intestines to expand and get in a lower the position in the abdomen. This then induces high pressure in the lower abdominal region, which results as stiffness on the front edge of the Pubis and the Ilium. This tension pulls the lower back from the inside of the abdomen.

The problem can be approached from the frontal myofascia tension lines and from the back lines.

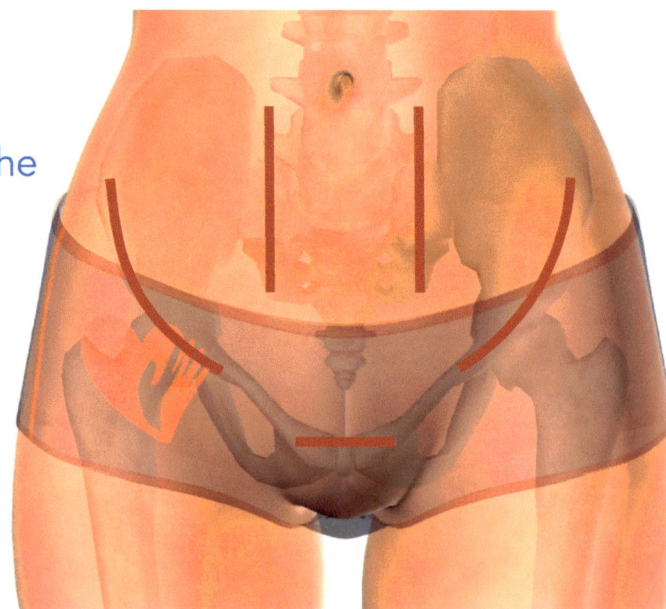

TIP!

Fast eating is the first reason for digestive stress! Not using enough saliva and swallowing chunks of food creates a large amount of gas in the intestines. They get heavier and in a lower position, which causes high pressure and high tension on the lower belly. Chew more to feel more saliva!

RELEASING TENSION ON THE ABDOMEN

Mechanism:

First work on the frontal part of the body. The abdominal region tension can be released by applying treatment along several myofascial tension lines that stretch from as up as the chin, down along the trunk, splitting down the two legs and ending in the toes.

There are several lines, as shown with the Green Lines. The treatment points are on bone edges marked in red. As always, start your treatments from the farthest points to release tension of:

1. The Ilium edge
2. The Pubis edge
3. The Rectus Abdominis

See Also:
Superficial Front Line - Anatomy Train
YangMing of foot meridian muscle - Jing jin

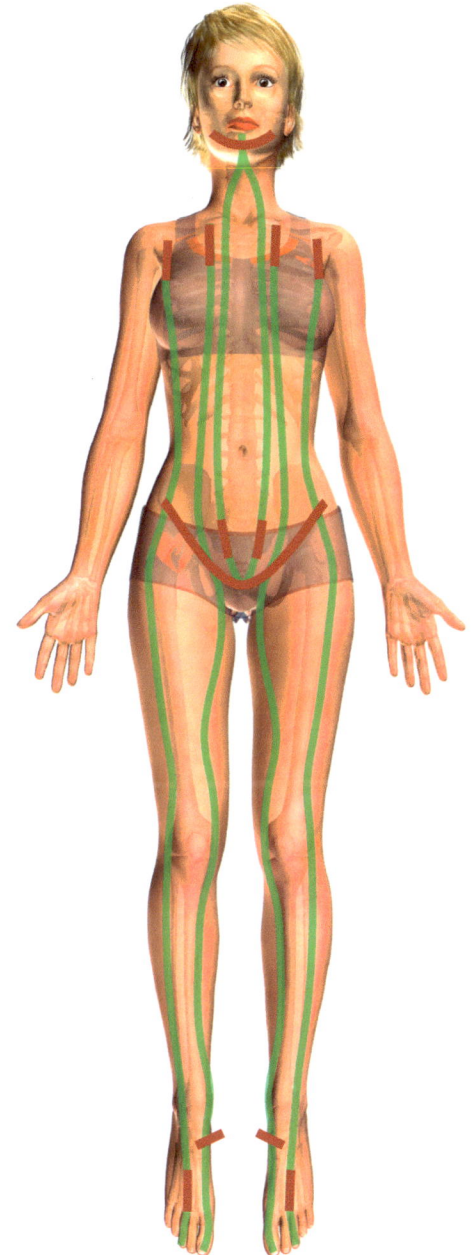

RELEASING TENSION ON THE ILIUM EDGE

To release tension on the Ilium edge, you must work on both feet and both sides of the upper chest before you touch the area itself.

Treatment: SCRATCHES

1. SCRATCH beneath the medial Malleolus
2. SCRATCH between Metatarsals

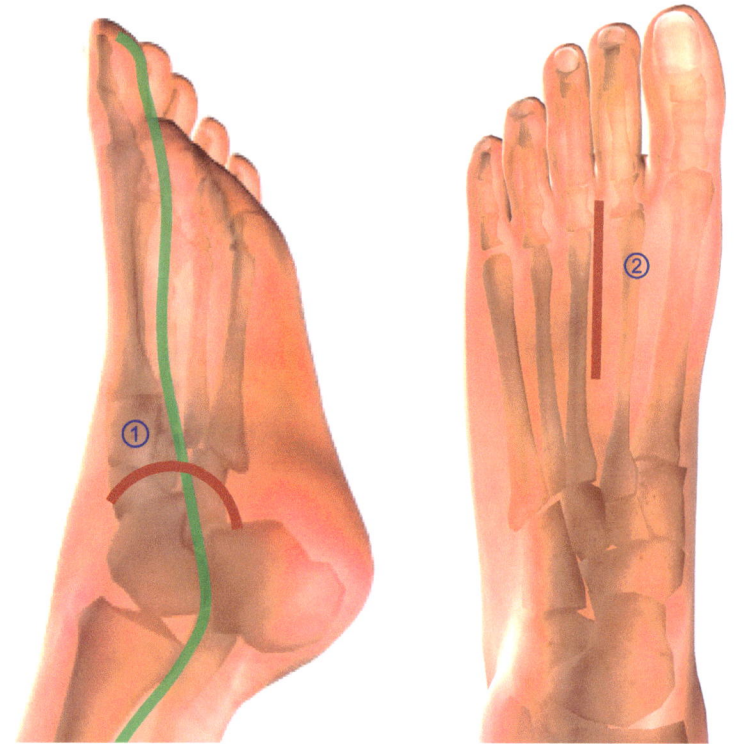

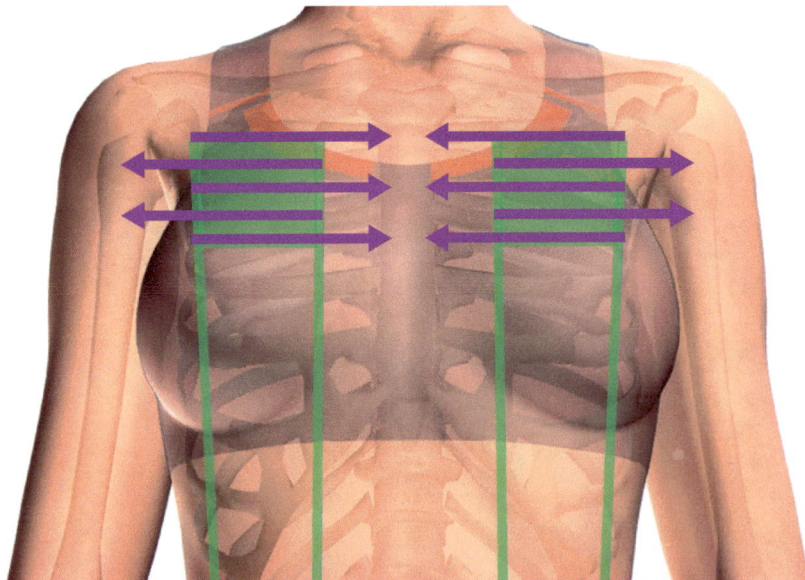

Treatment: SLIDE

1. Imagine the green square, and SLIDE it to lateral

Treatment: SLIDE

1. Touch the edge of Ilium and SLIDE it toward the inside

Don't push in strongly to the abdominal organs.

⚠️ If your patient is reluctant to this technique, you can teach them how to perform it by themselves.

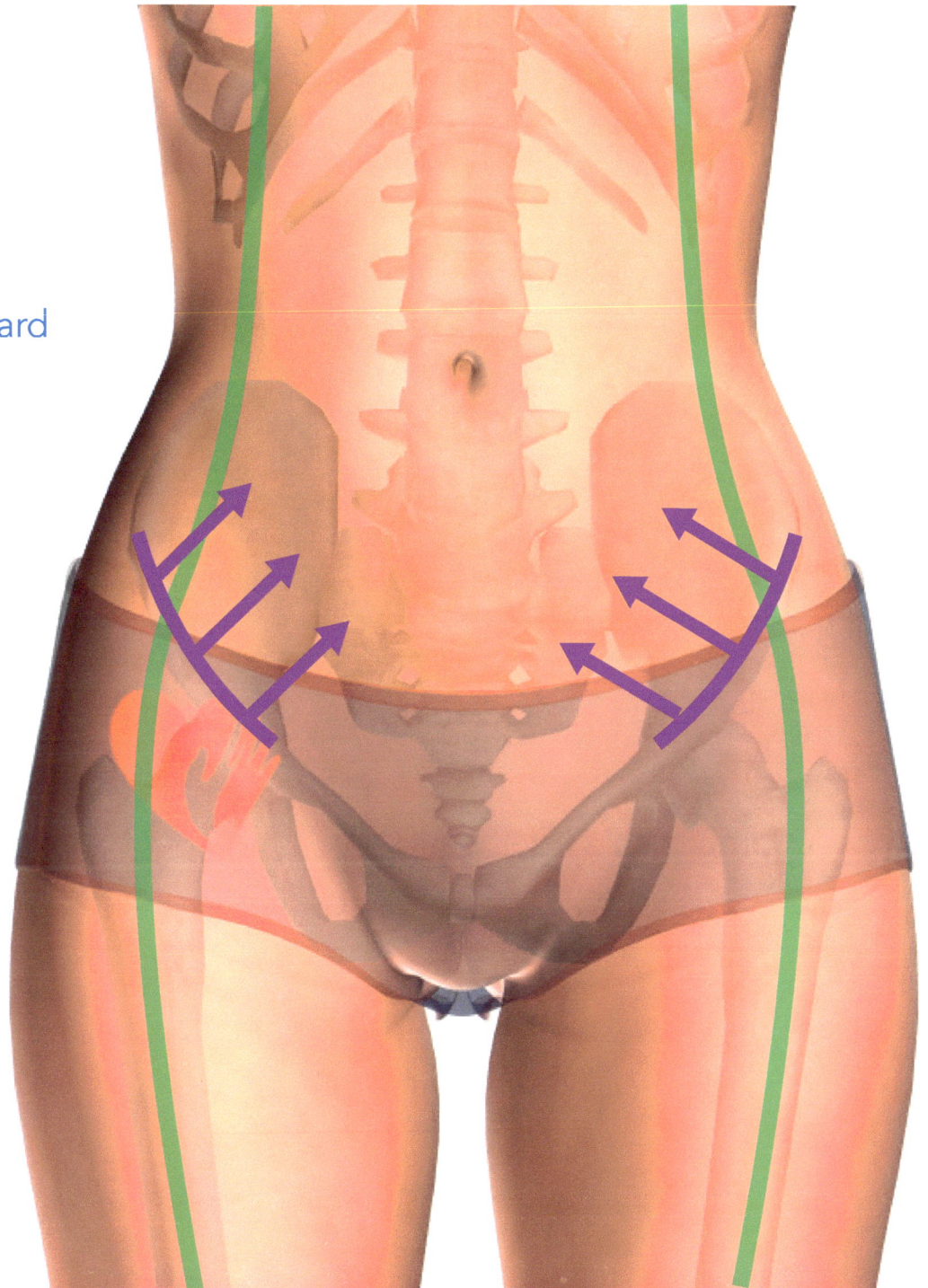

RELEASING TENSION ON PUBIS EDGE

Before you work on the Pubis edge, you must start by releasing the tension on the chin.

Treatment: SCRATCHES

1. SCRATCH the chin along the red lines to release sticking myofascia on the chin edge.

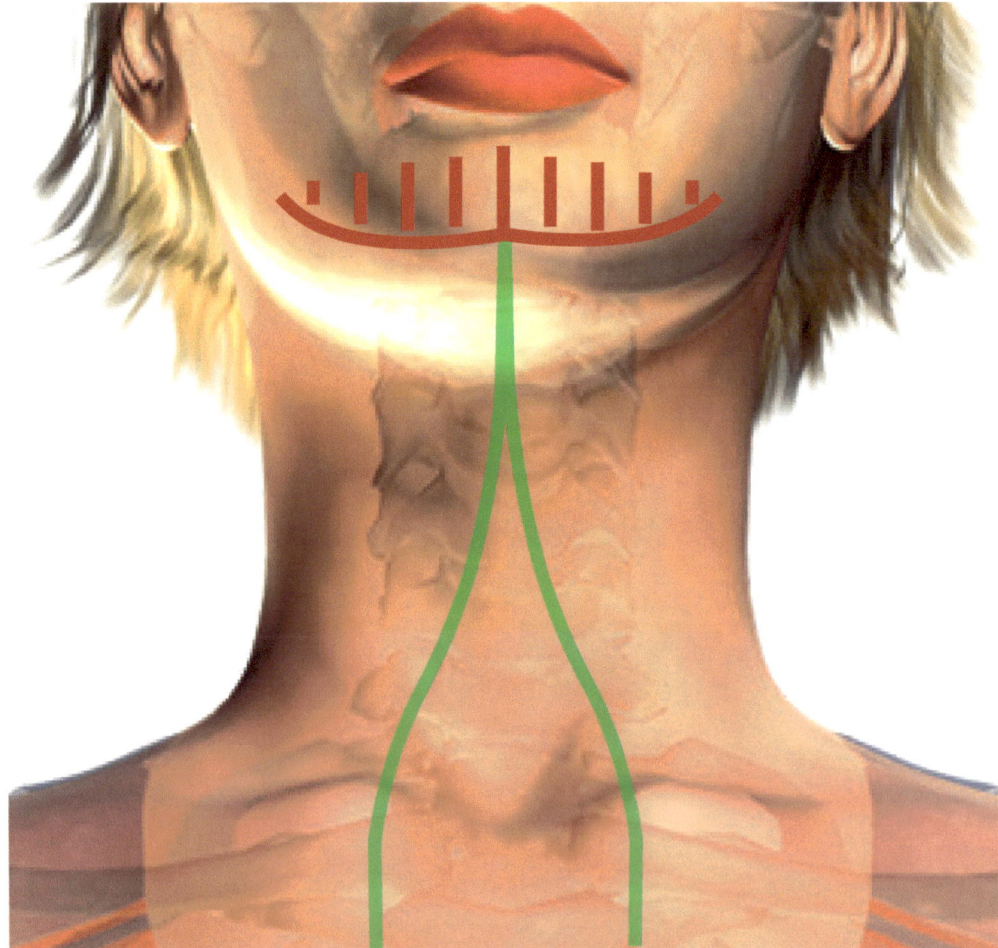

Treatment:

1. Touch the edge of the Ilium and SLIDE it toward the inside

Don't push in strongly on the abdominal organs.

This area is considered very private on ALL patients. Carefully explain what you will be doing and ask for permission FIRST.

Make sure that the entire area is fully covered with cloth before performing your treatment.

If the patient is reluctant, simply skip this treatment.

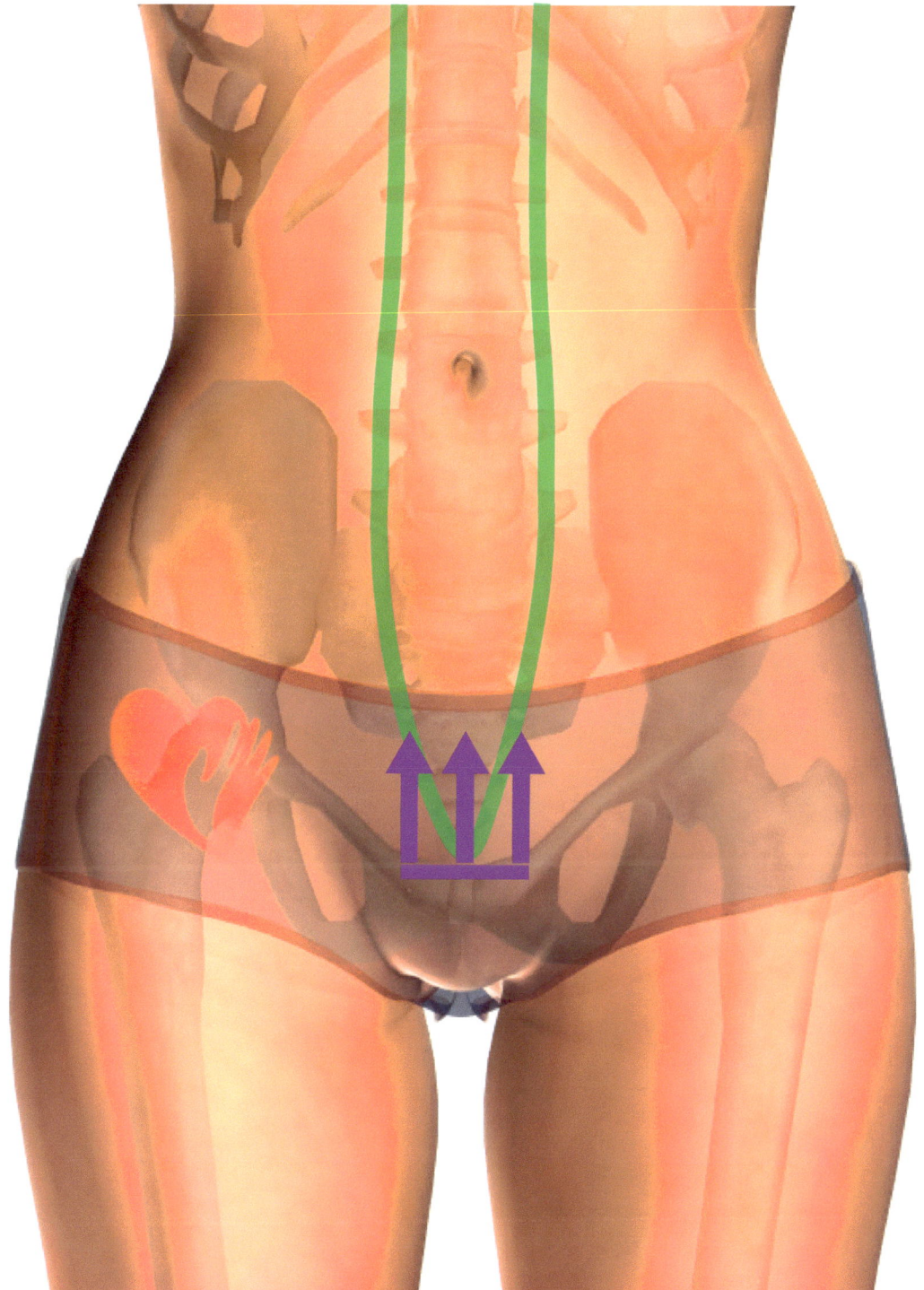

RELEASING TENSION ON THE RECTUS ABDOMINIS

Treatment: SLIDE

1. Look for the lateral edge of the Rectus Abdominis and SLIDE it to medial

⚠ Don't push in strongly on the abdominal organs. You may notice tensed lines (purple lines) after starting. SLIDE them.

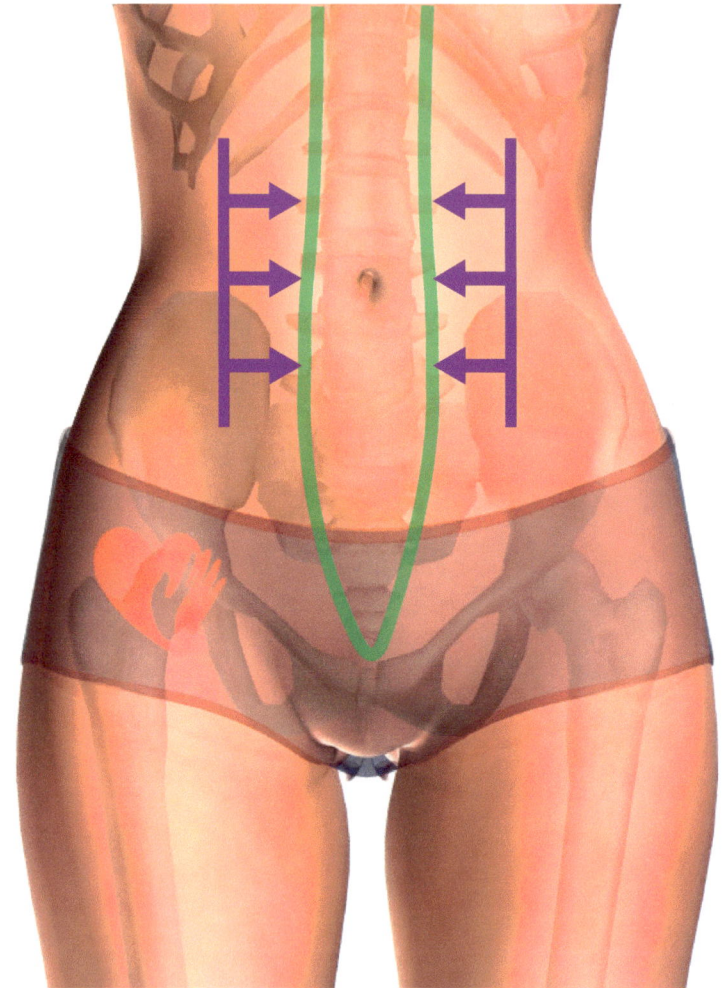

TIP!
When the abdominal tension is released, many patients mention that they feel their hips are more opened and that they get a much better sleep.

RELEASING BACK TENSION

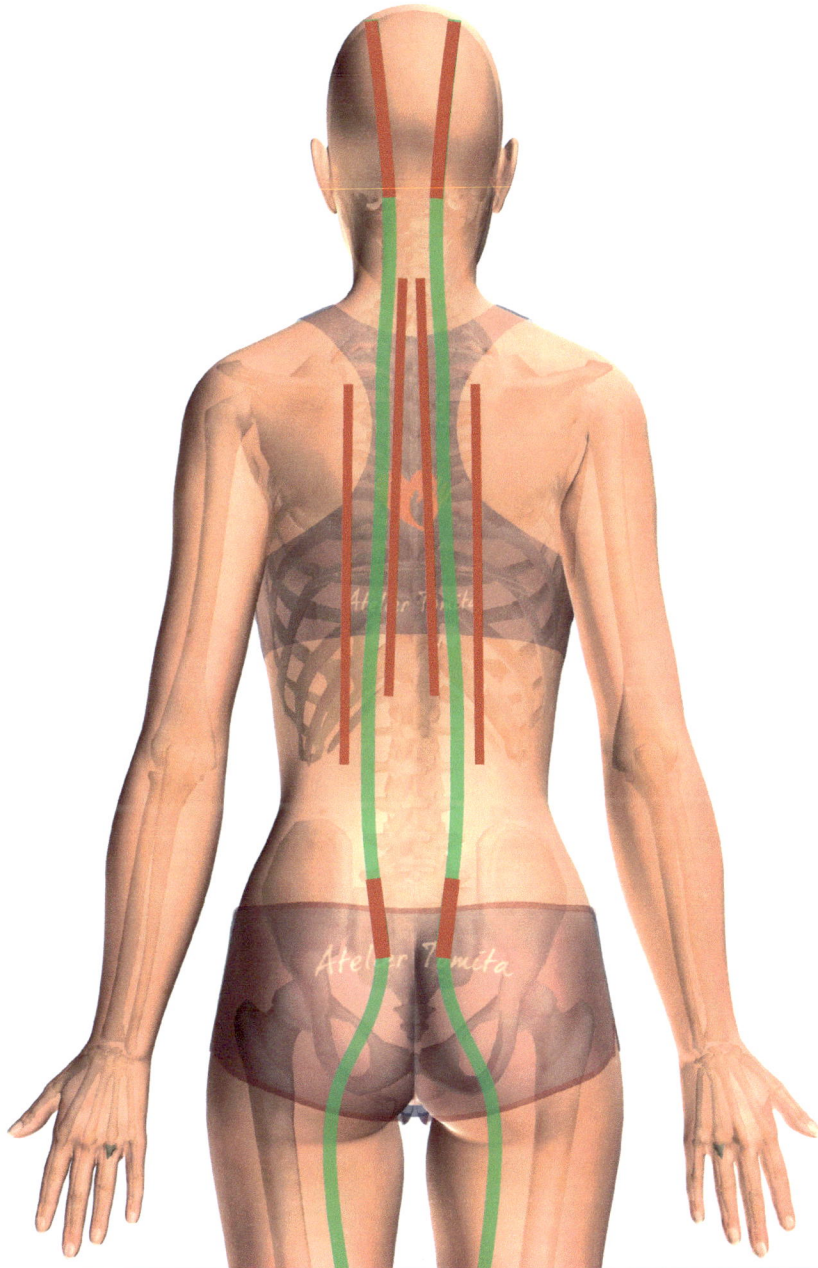

Mechanism:

The second part of your work in releasing abdominal tension is to apply treatment along the back myofascial tension connecting lines.

There are two main lines, attached on the skull at one end, which go down to the feet, as shown with the Green Lines.

Tension at the lower back causes problems mainly on the shoulders, neck and head.

The treatment points are marked in red.

See also:
Superficial Back Line - Anatomy Train
TaiYang of foot meridian muscle - Jing jin

RELEASING TENSION ON THE ERECTOR SPINAE

Releasing tension on the Erector Spinae is a long and minute process. You have to apply your treatment on the back of the head first and go down from the start of the neck to the lower back. These two techniques demand patience and minuteness. Pay attention to the result of each maneuver.

Treatment: SCRATCHES

1. SCRATCH around the red area

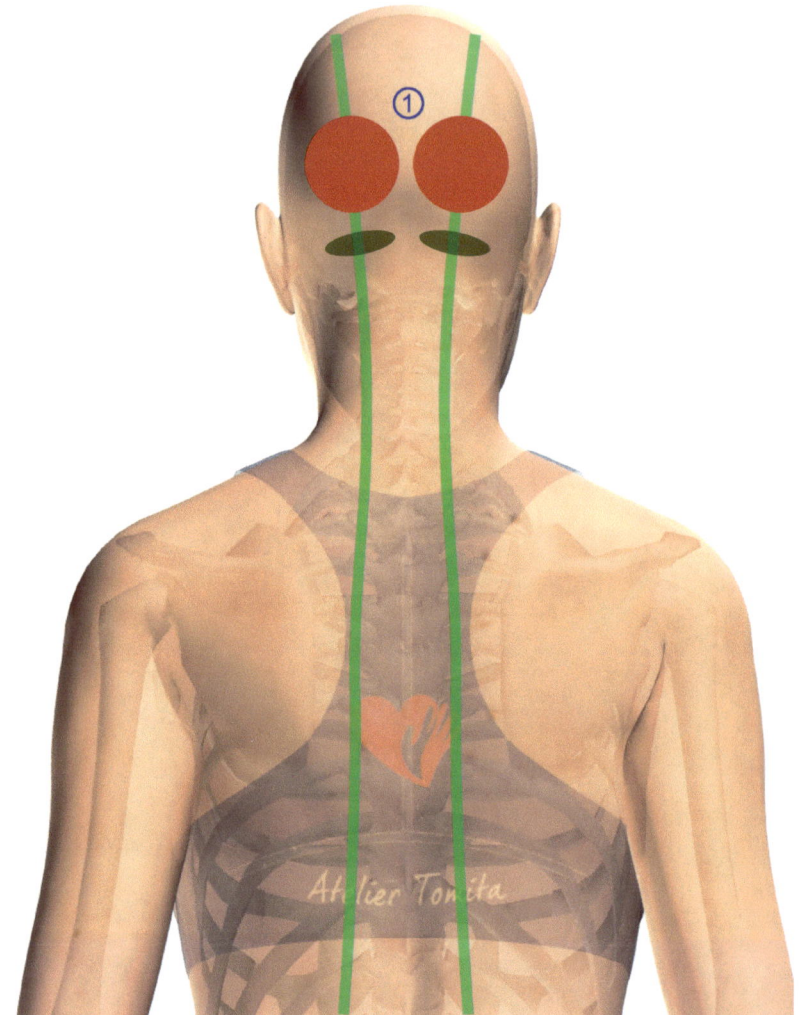

TIP!

If you touch simultaneously the lower green point on the upper neck while performing your treatment, you may feel the tightening tension decrease with the treatment.

The way to care: SCRATCHES

1. SCRATCH along the red line and SLIDE it to lateral
2. SCRATCH the lateral side of the Erector Spinae and SLIDE it to medial

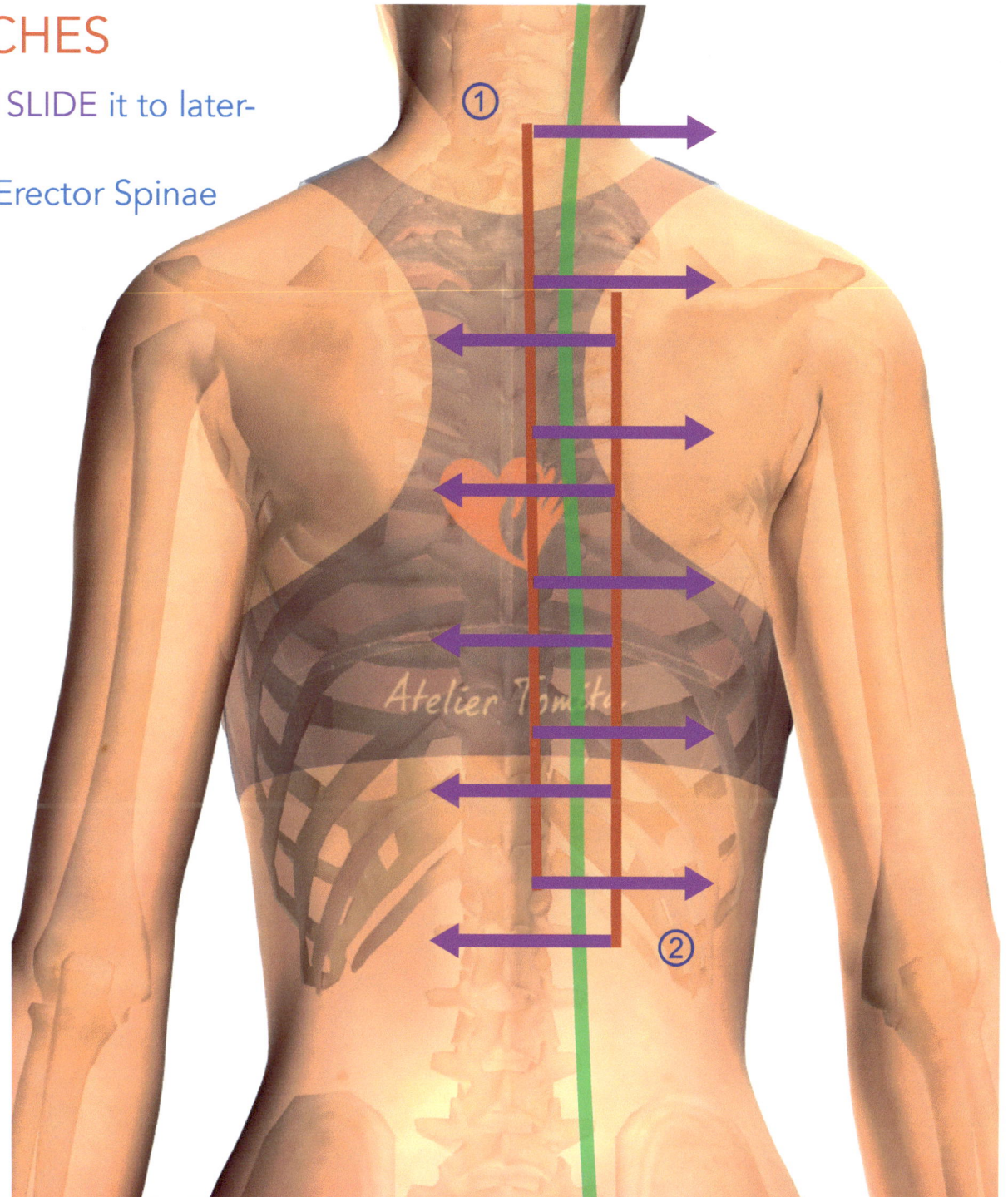

①

②

RELEASING TENSION ON THE INTERCOSTAL MUSCLE

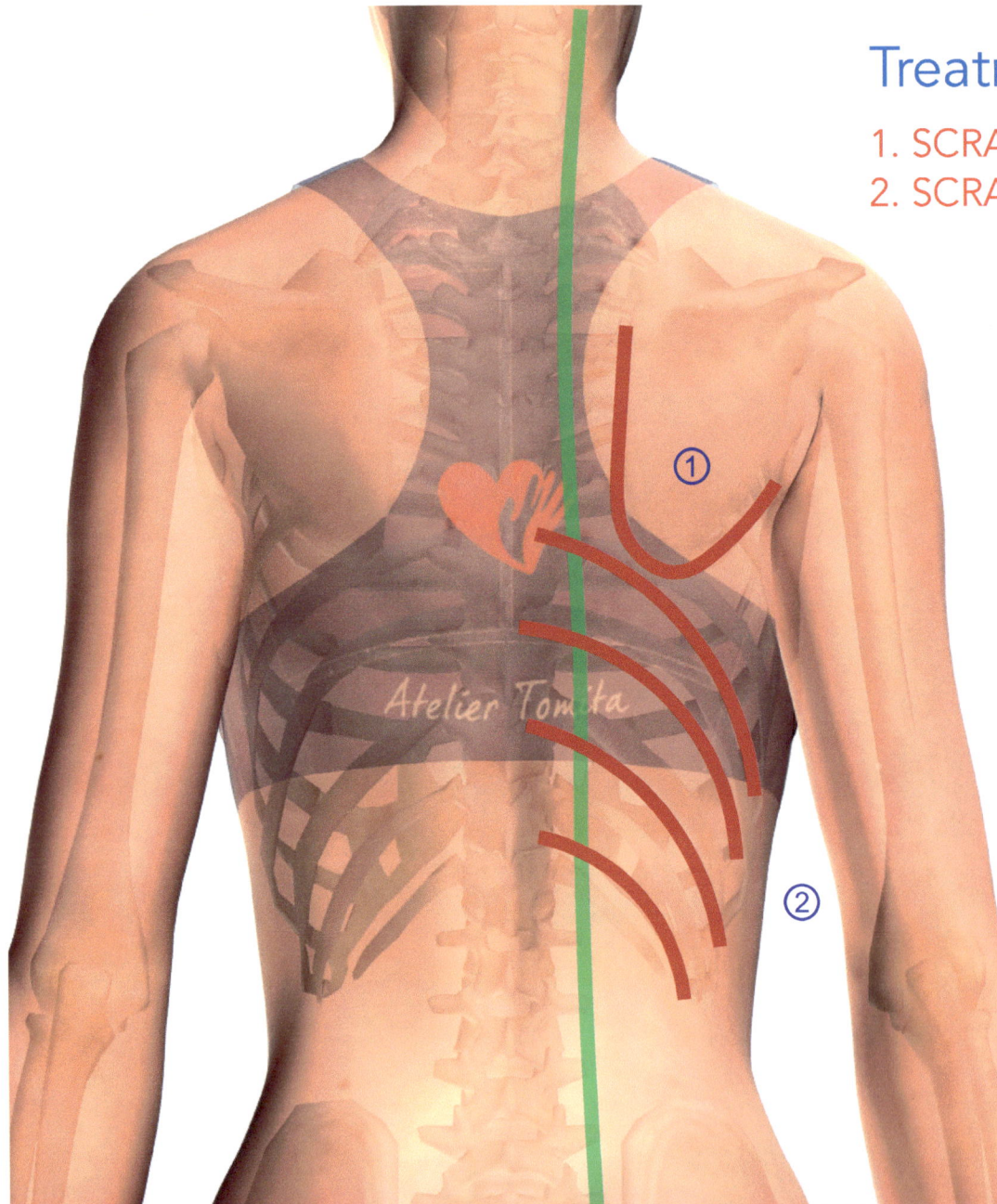

Treatment: SCRATCHES

1. SCRATCH the medial edge of the Scapula
2. SCRATCH the inferior edge of each rib bone

①

②

⚠️ SCRATCHING the rib cage can be ticklish. Tell your patient the purpose of the treatment before you start.

Atelier Tomita

RELEASING TENSION ON SACRUM

Treatment: SCRATCHES

1. SCRATCH along the hollow of the Sacrum and SLIDE it to lateral
2. SCRATCH along the hollow lateral side of the Sacrum and slide it to lateral

These points are close to the Anus and Genitals. A polite explanation is necessary before the treatment.

Check that the entire area is properly covered with cloth before you start.

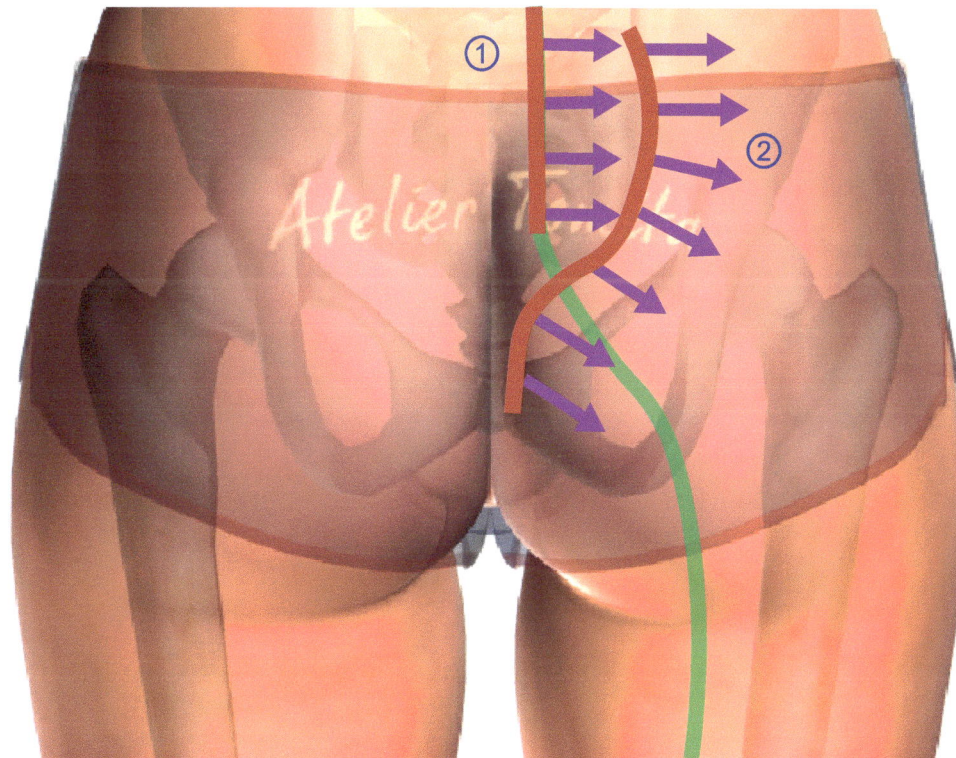

EVALUATION

1. Can you explain the mechanism and causes of abdominal and inner back pain?

2. Can you explain the different areas of treatment necessary to release abdominal tension?

3. Can you explain the different areas of treatment necessary to release back tension?

4. Can you perform the Erector Spinae tension release technique?

5. What advice can you give to your patient to prevent abdominal and back pain?

NOTES

HEAD AND EARS

OUTLINE

1. Understanding Head tension
1. Releasing scalp skin tension
   - Releasing back scalp skin tension
   - Releasing side scalp skin tension
2. Releasing ears stiffness
3. Releasing facial tension

UNDERSTANDING HEAD TENSION

Mechanism:

The head is a terminal of myofascial tensions. The tensions come up from the back, the chest, from all around the trunk. There are several specific myofascial tension connection lines on head, and the tension spreads stiffly all over the scalp, the ears and the face. Your patient might not directly feel pain around those areas, but it is crucial to release these tensions if you diagnose them, as they are connected with the whole body.

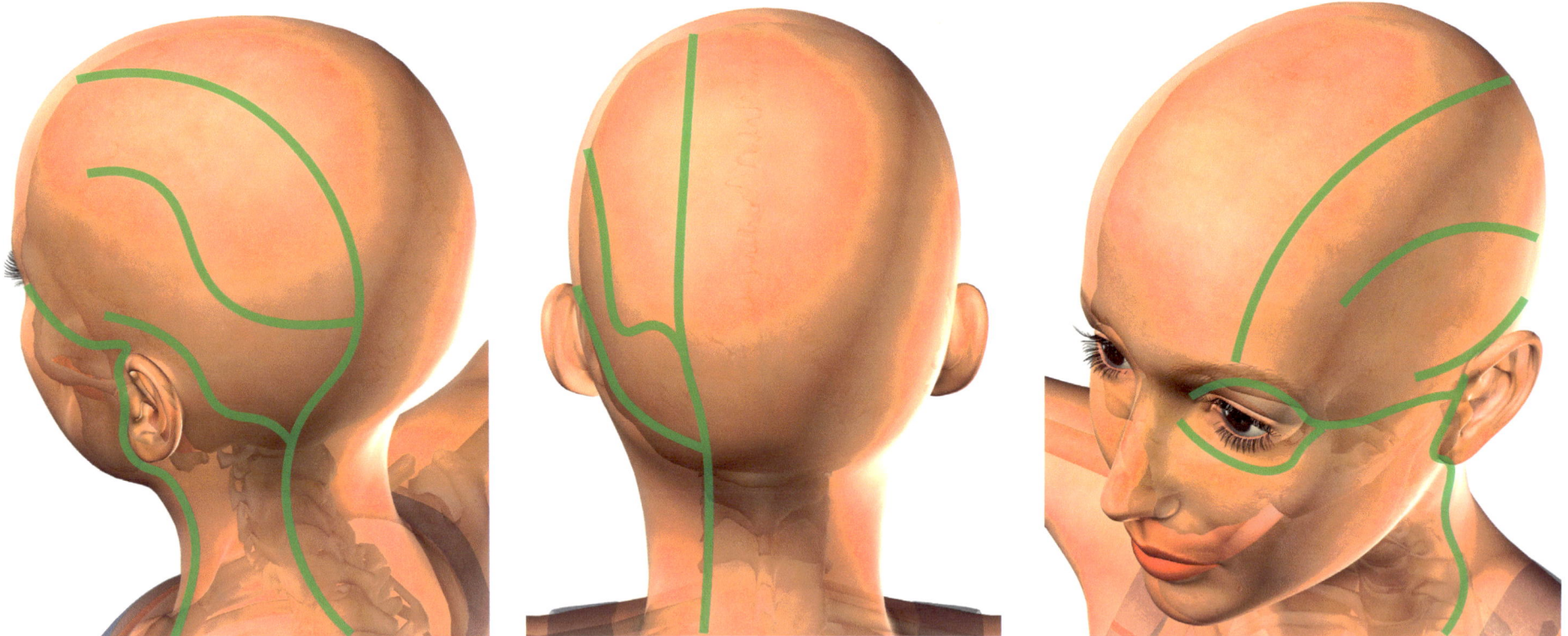

RELEASING SCALP SKIN TENSION

Mechanism:

The head is not perfect sphere, it's convexoconcave. The myofascial tension is concentrated around the convex and the concave areas. Here we have purposely exaggerated those area on the images, to facilitate the understanding of the mechanisms.
There are two main myofascial tension lines on the head, one of which splits into three branches.

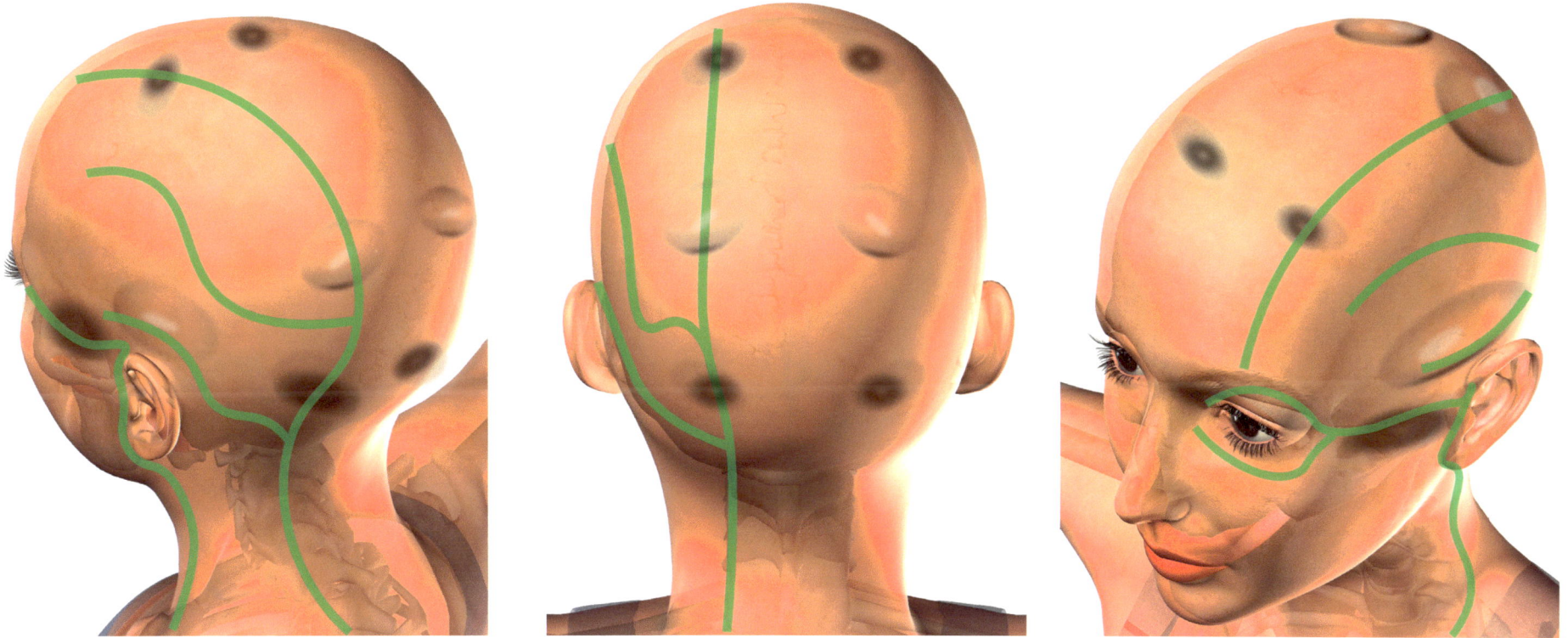

See also:
Superficial Back Line/Deep Front Line - Anatomy Train
TaiYang/ShaoYang of foot meridian muscle - Jing jin

RELEASING BACK SCALP SKIN TENSION

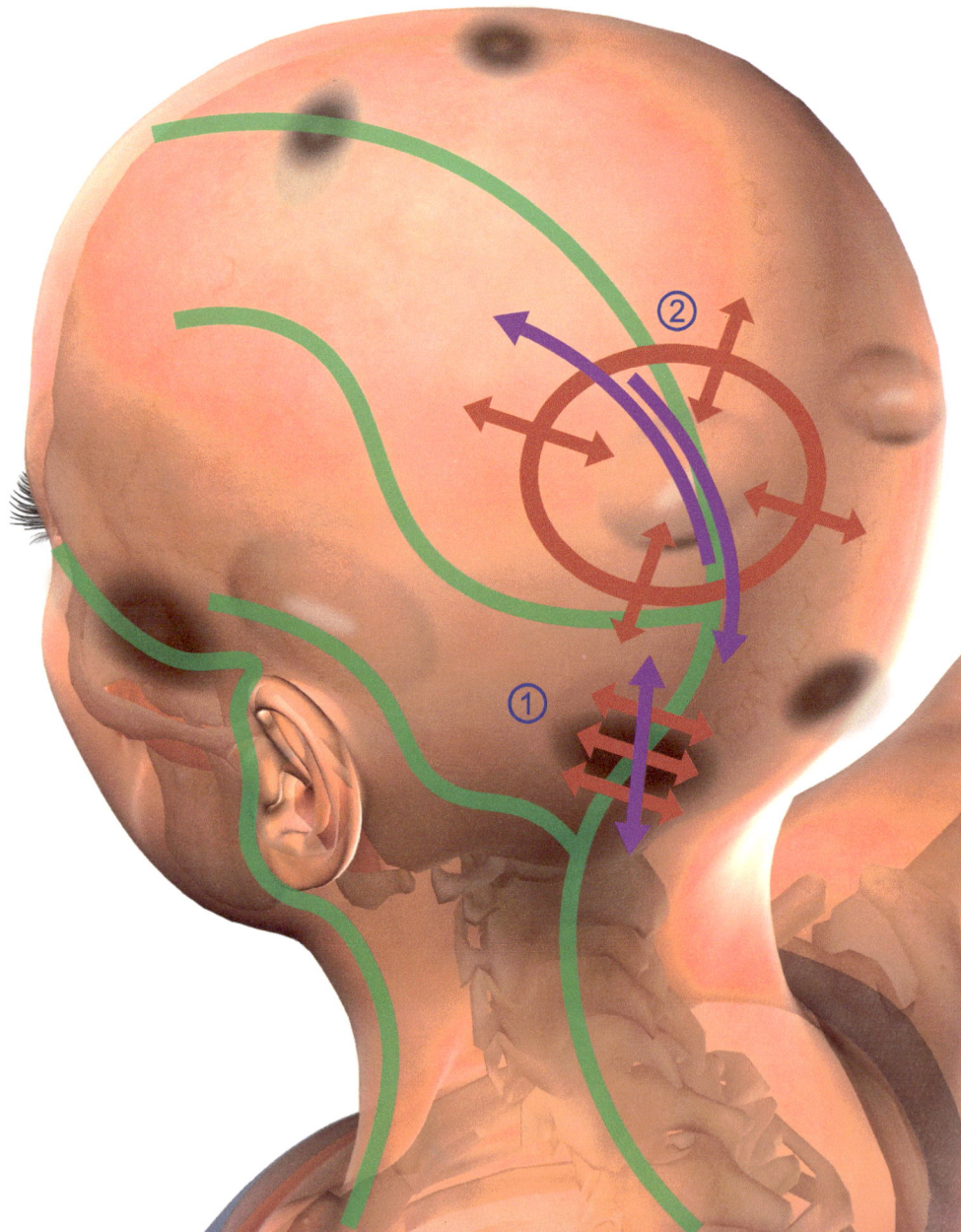

The way to care: SCRATCHES

1. SCRATCH the concave spot at back of the head and SLIDE the skin on top of it
2. SCRATCH around the convex area at the back of the head and SLIDE the skin on top of it

⚠️ Some patients don't want you to touch their head, for several reasons. You can teach them how to perform the SCRATCHES themselves, or, if they prefer a more gentle approach, the STROKES technique.

The way to care: STROKES

1. STROKE the back of the head upward as shown with the Blue Arrows

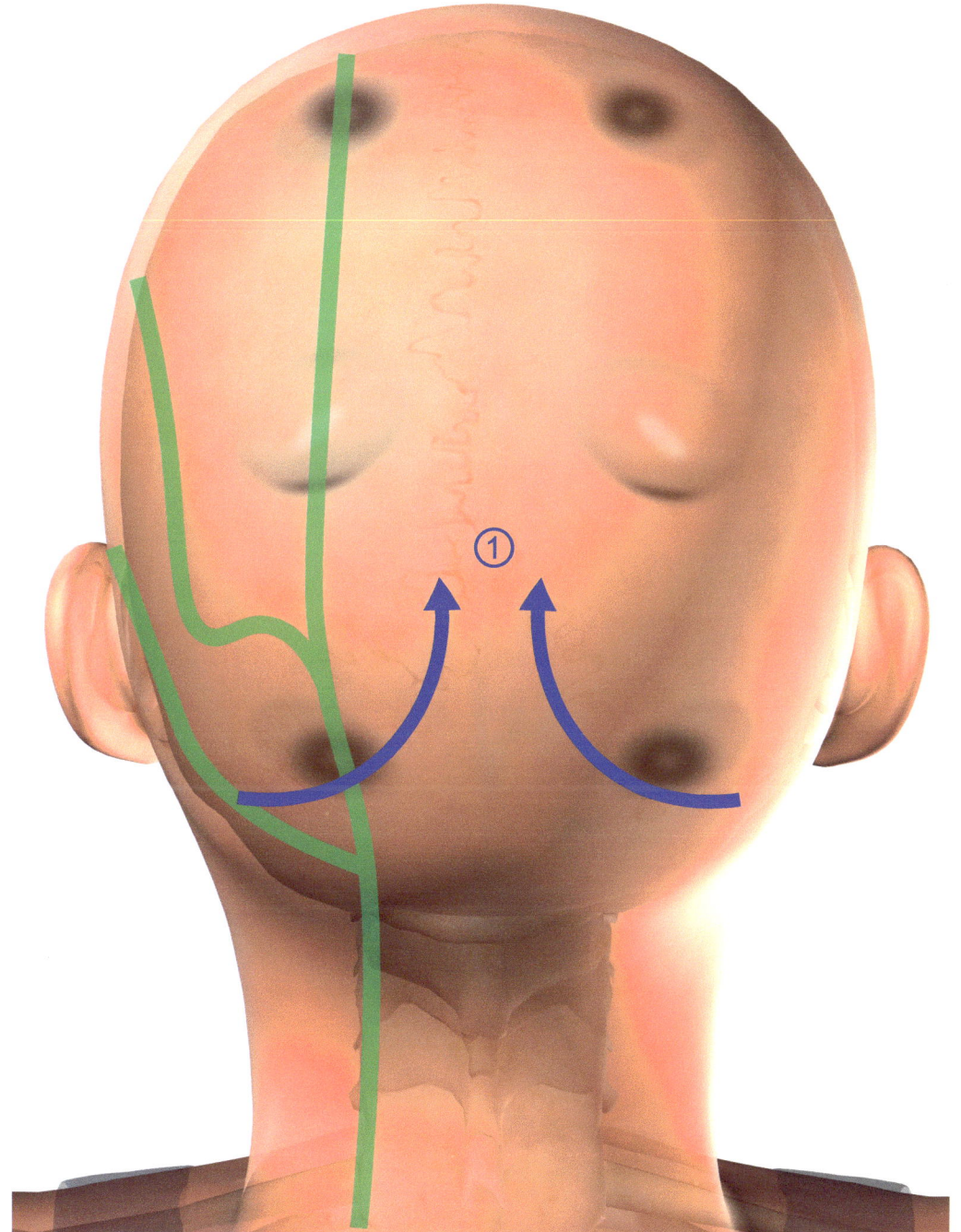

RELEASING SIDE SCALP SKIN TENSION

Treatment: SCRATCHES

1. SCRATCH the convex area at side of the head and SLIDE the skin on top of it
2. SLIDE in circles the convex point at side head

Again, you can teach reluctant patients how to perform the SCRATCHES themselves, or, if they prefer a more gentle approach, the STROKES technique.

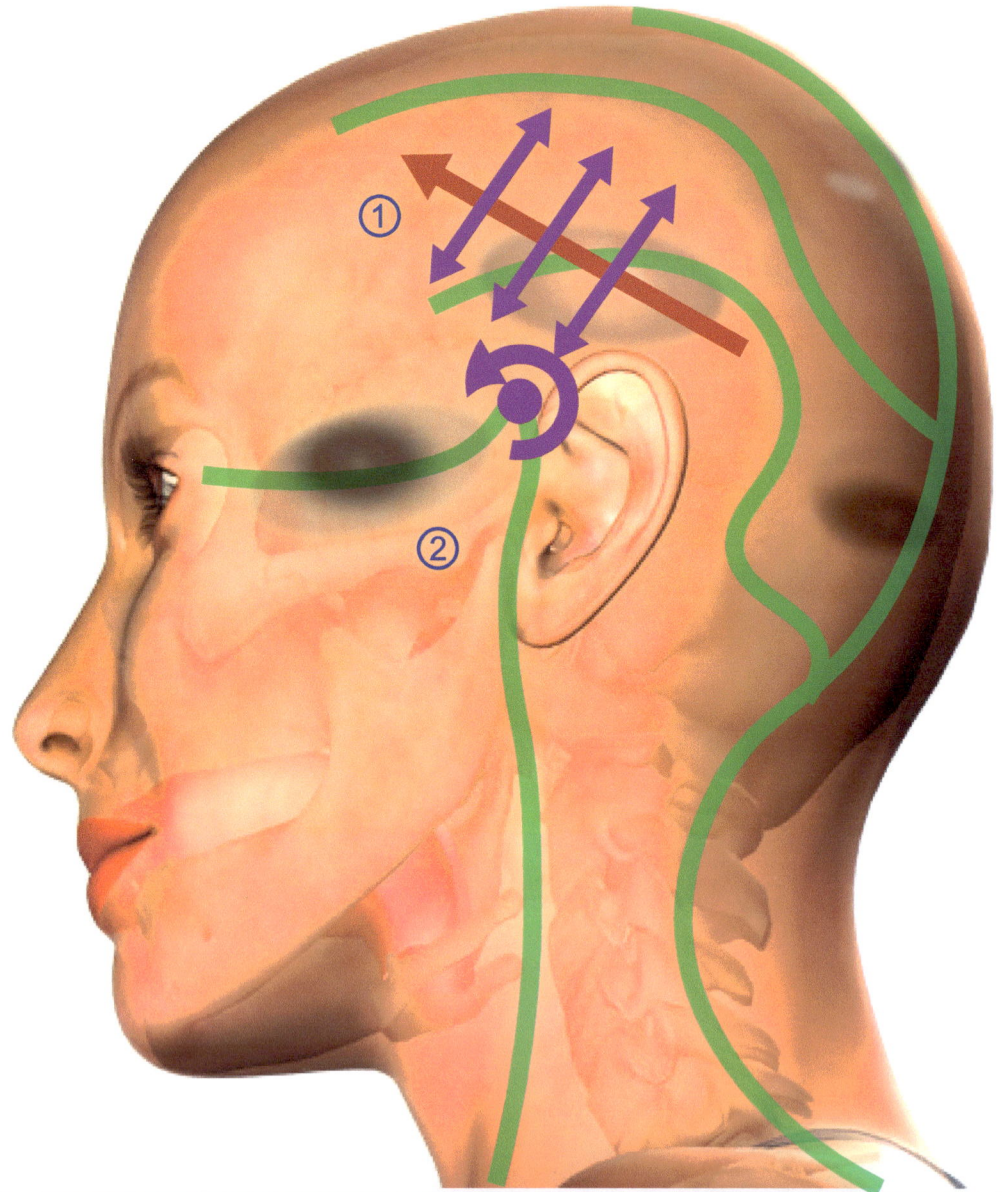

Treatment: STROKES

1. STROKE the side head upward

This method is very gentle and can be taught to the patient as self-care maintenance.

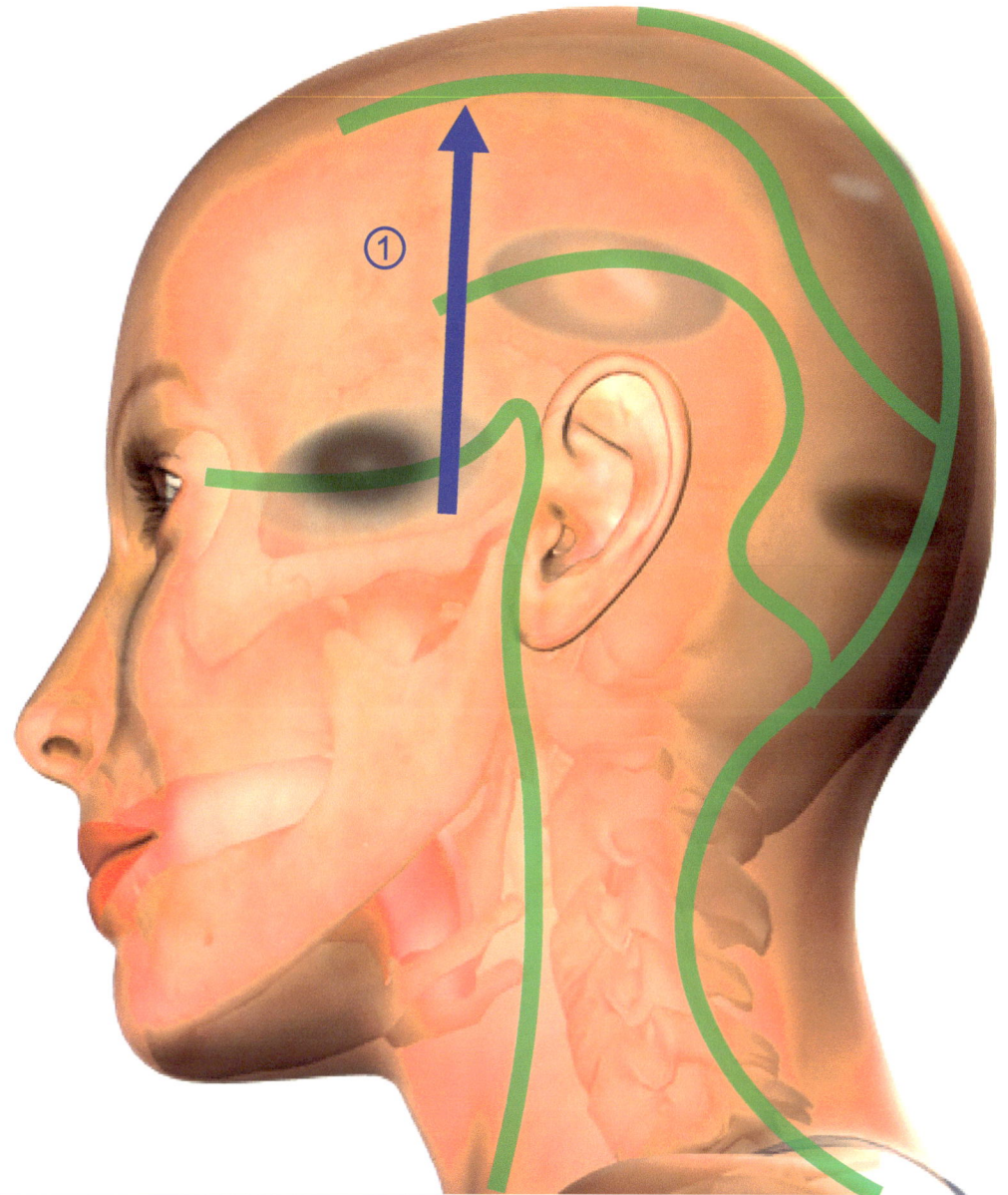

RELEASING EARS STIFFNESS

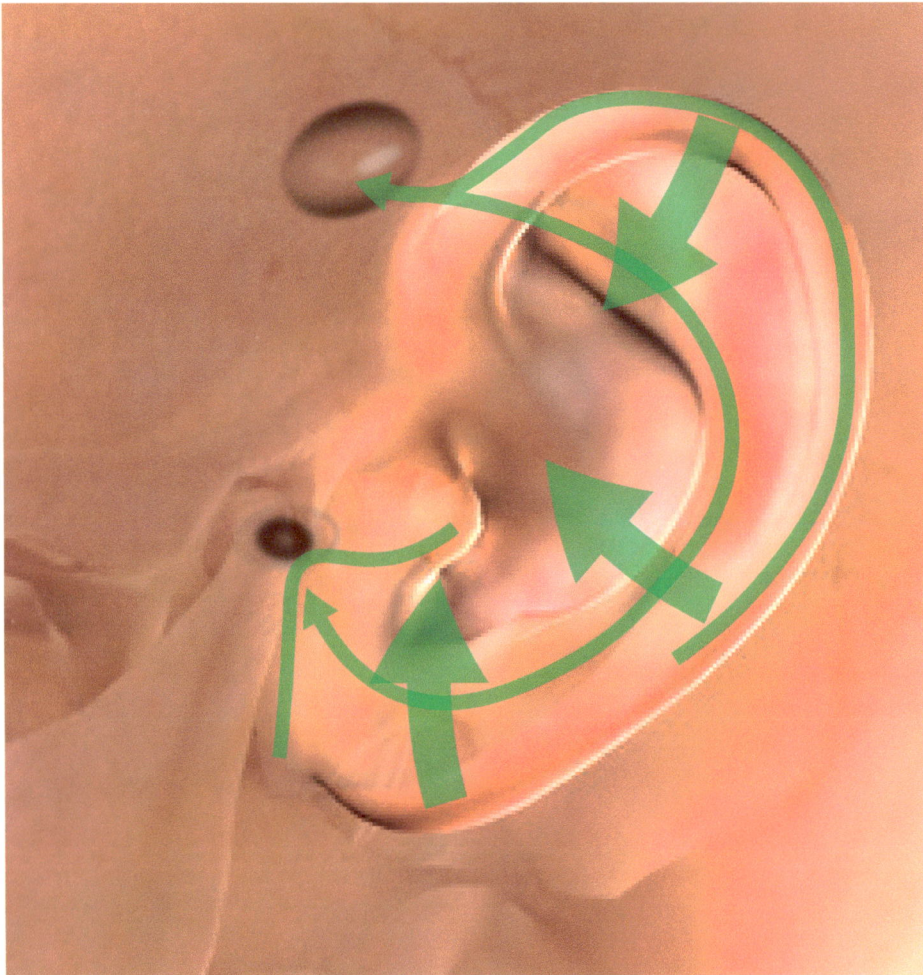

Mechanism:

The ear is one of the most distal part of the body, like the fingers and toes. It seems like the terminal of the entire myofascial tension. Tension is concentrated along the shape of the ear, as shown with the Green Lines, and this makes the ear stiff and shrink.

See also:
Deep Front Line - Anatomy Train
ShaoYang of hand/foot meridian muscle - Jing jin
Note: There are no details in these references, but they show the myofascial connection on the side of the head.

Treatment: PULLING

1. PULL out the upper helix to lateral by twisting the ear
2. PULL out the concha of auricle to lateral by twisting the ear
3. PULL out the cavity of concha to lateral by twisting the ear
4. Twist the Tragus

⚠ This might hurt at first, so WARN your patient before starting and perform the technique very gently.

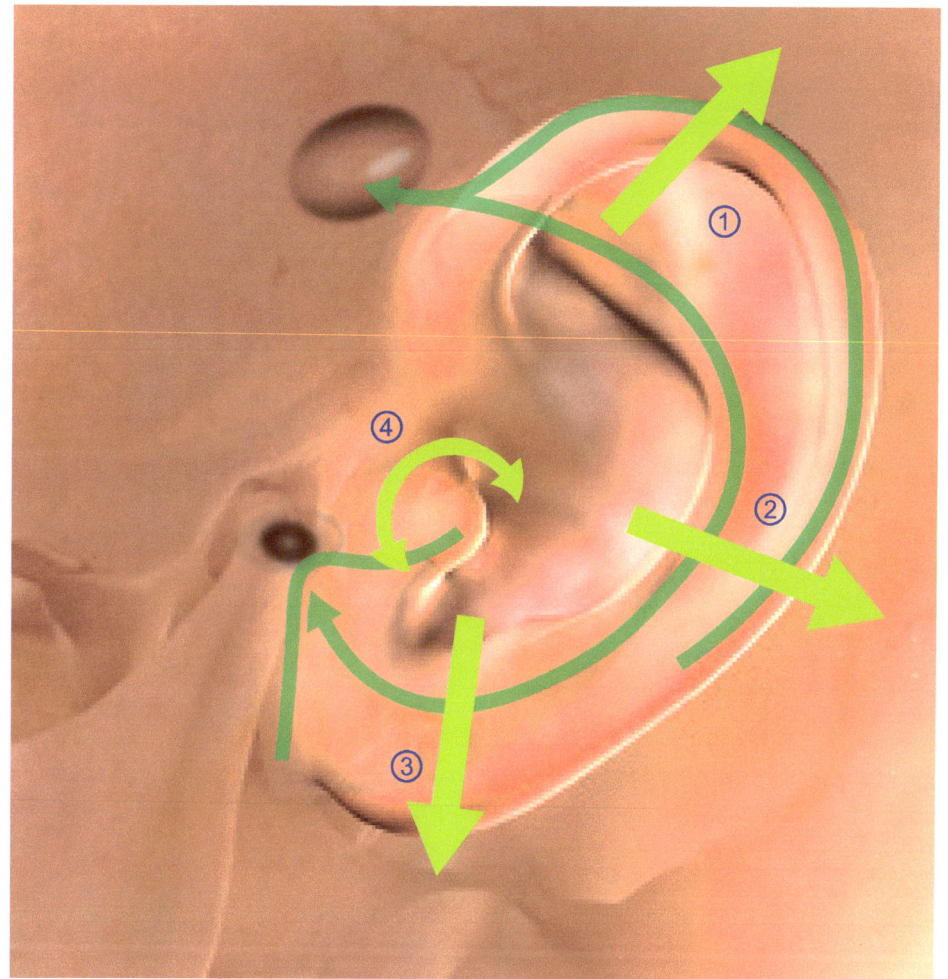

TIP!

A sudden strong PULL will NOT work. Take your time and gradually add gentle PULLING strength. After the treatment, the ear will become much softer and feel hot.

RELEASING FACIAL TENSION

Mechanism:

There are 2 major myofascial tensions lines on the cheeks. One comes up from the chest, and the other from jaw joints. Both of them are sticking at the inferior edge of the Zygomatic bone, as shown with the Green Line.
The treatment points are marked in red.

⚠️ Remember that the skin on the face is thinner and more delicate than other parts of the body. Use a slightly thicker cloth on this area for the SCRATCHING method.

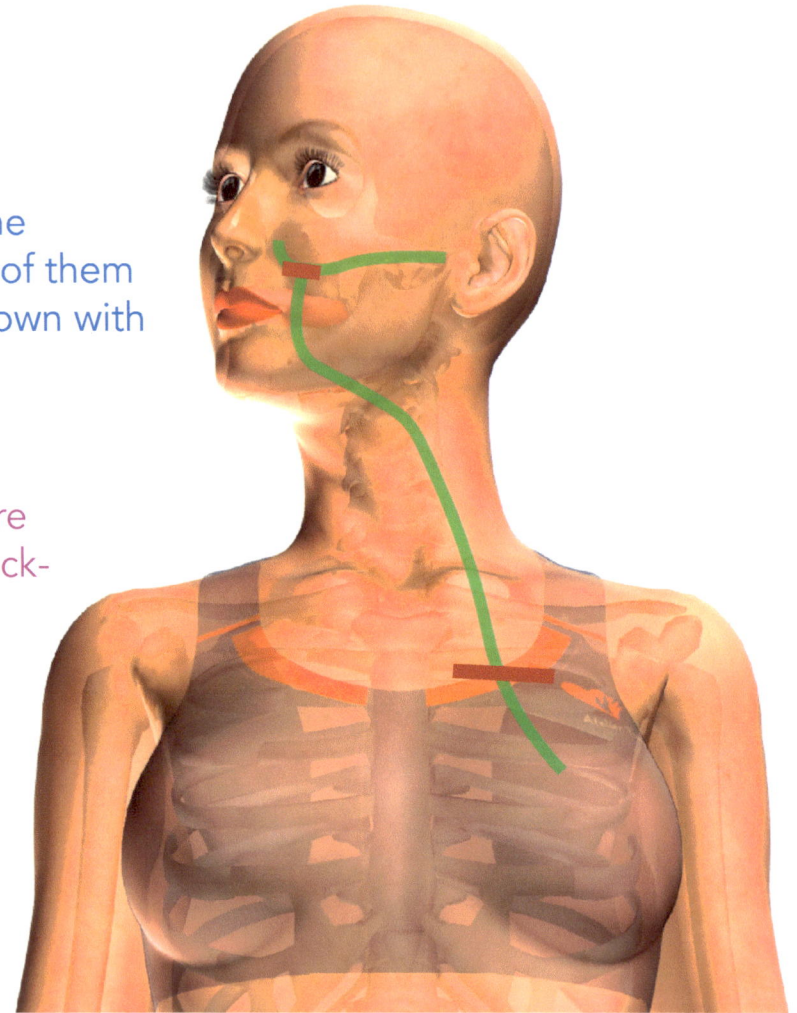

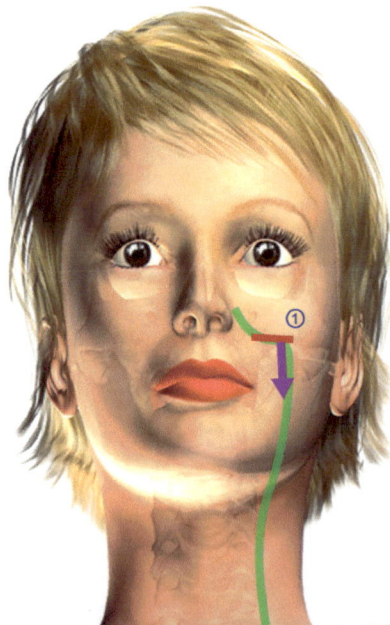

Treatment: SCRATCHES

1. Dig the inferior edge of the Zygomatic bone and SLIDE it to inferior

Treatment: SCRATCHES

1. SCRATCH the inferior edge of the Clavicle and rib bones and SLIDE to lateral

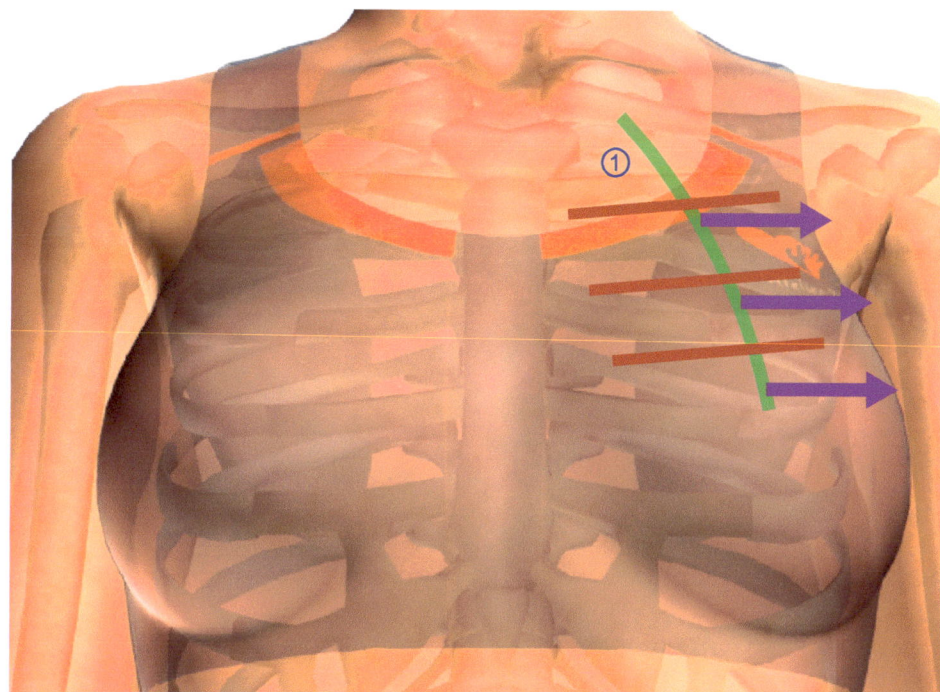

Treatment: STROKES

1. STROKE the superior/inferior both edges of the Clavicle to medial

The STROKES technique can be used if the patient feels too much pain. It is also an easily performed self-care method to teach to your patient for maintenance.

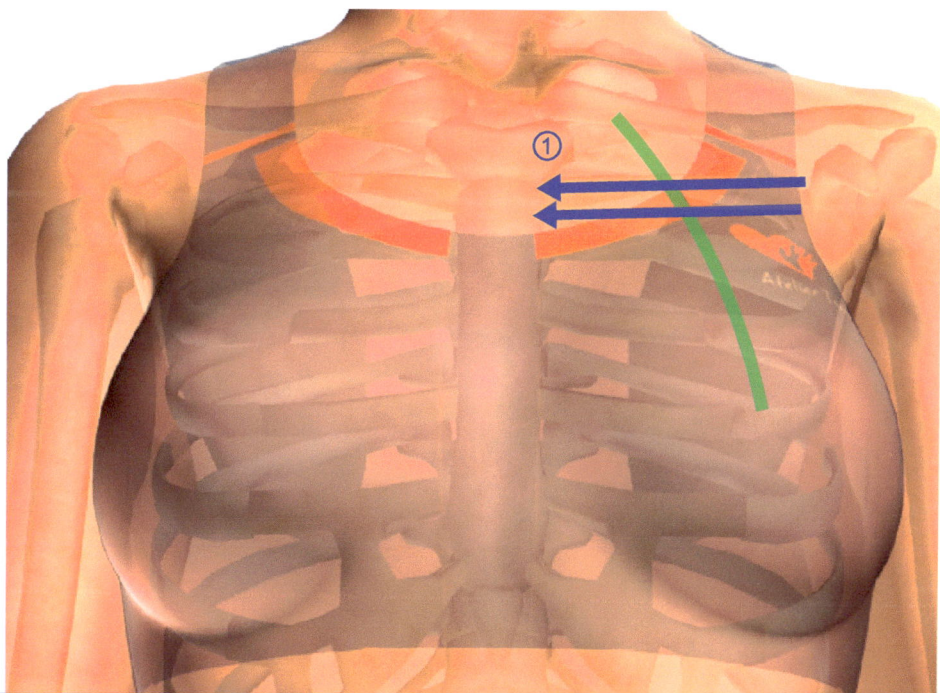

EVALUATION

1. Can you explain the mechanism of the head myofascial tension?

2. Can you release head skin tension?

3. Can you release ear tension?

4. Can you release facial tension?

5. What self-care techniques can you teach your patient?

NOTES

Author
Norio Tomita
info@ateliertomita.com

Designer and Editor
Christine Lavoie-Gagnon

Publisher
CLAGA
www.claga.net

2017